Managing Diabetic Nephropathies in Clinical Practice

George L. Bakris • Allison Hahr
Romesh Khardori • Daisuke Koya
Mark Molitch • Friedrich C. Prischl
Guntram Schernthaner •
Bijin Thajudeen

Managing Diabetic Nephropathies in Clinical Practice

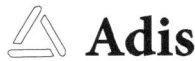

George L. Bakris
Department of Medicine
The University of Chicago
Chicago, Illinois
USA

Allison Hahr
Feinberg School of Medicine
Northwestern University
Chicago, Illinois
USA

Romesh Khardori
East Virginia Medical School
Norfolk, Virginia
USA

Daisuke Koya
Kanazawa Medical University
Uchinada
Japan

Mark Molitch
Feinberg School of Medicine
Northwestern University
Chicago, Illinois
USA

Friedrich C. Prischl
Klinikum Wels-Grieskirchen
Wels
Austria

Guntram Schernthaner
Rudolfstiftung Hospital-Vienna
Wien
Austria

Bijin Thajudeen
University of Arizona
Tuscon, Arizona
USA

ISBN 978-3-319-08872-3   ISBN 978-3-319-08873-0   (eBook)
DOI 10.1007/978-3-319-08873-0

Library of Congress Control Number: 2016944004

Printed on acid-free paper

This Adis imprint is published by Springer Nature
The registered company is Springer International Publishing AG Switzerland

Author Biographies

George L. Bakris, MD, Hon. DSc, FASH, FASN, FAHA, is a Professor of Medicine and Director at the ASH Comprehensive Hypertension Center, The University of Chicago Medicine, Chicago, Illinois. Dr. Bakris received his medical degree from the Rosalind Franklin School of Medicine and completed residency in *Internal Medicine* at the Mayo Graduate School of Medicine where he also completed a research fellowship in *Physiology and Biophysics*. He then completed fellowships in *Nephrology* and *Clinical Pharmacology* at the University of Chicago. From 1988 to 1991, he served as Director of Renal Research at the Ochsner Clinic and had faculty appointments in the Departments of Medicine and Physiology at Tulane University School of Medicine. He later was Professor and Vice Chairman of *Preventive Medicine and Director of the Rush University Hypertension Center* in Chicago from 1993 until 2006. *Currently*, he is a *Professor of Medicine* and *Director of the ASH Comprehensive Hypertension Center* in the Department of Medicine at the University of Chicago Medicine.

Dr. Bakris has published over 700 peer-reviewed articles and book chapters in the areas of diabetic kidney disease, hypertension, and progression of nephropathy. He is the Editor or Co-Editor of 20 books in the areas of kidney disease progression and diabetes as well as the new edition of *Hypertension: A Companion to Braunwald's The Heart*. Additionally, he is an Associate Editor of the *International Textbook of Cardiology*. He was a member of the NIH National High Blood Pressure Education Program Working

Group on Hypertension and Renal Disease (1994). He also serves as a special government expert to the Cardio-renal Advisory Board of the FDA and to CMS. He was a co-principal investigator on the NIH Clinical Research training grant for clinical research (K30) (1999–2004). He chaired the *first* National Kidney Foundation Consensus report on blood pressure and impact on renal disease progression (2000). He has also served on many national guideline committees including: The Joint National Committee Writing Groups VI & 7 (1997, 2003), the JNC 7 executive committee (2003), the American Diabetes Association Clinical Practice Guideline Committee (2002–2004), the National Kidney Foundation (K-DOQI) Blood Pressure Guideline committee (2002–2004 and 2013), and (K-DOQI) Diabetes Guideline committee (2003–2005 and 2014). Dr. Bakris is the past-president of the American College of Clinical Pharmacology (2000–2002) and the American Society of Hypertension (ASH). He is the current Editor-in-Chief, *Am J Nephrology*, Editor-in-Chief *Up-to-Date,* Nephrology section, Hypertension Section Editor *Up-to-Date,* and Assoc. Ed of *Diabetes Care.* He serves on more than 18 editorial boards including *Nephrology, Dialysis & Transplant, Hypertension, J Hypertension* and *J American Soc. Hypertension.*

Allison J. Hahr, MD, is an Assistant Professor at Northwestern University Feinberg School of Medicine in Chicago, Illinois. She trained in internal medicine and endocrinology at Northwestern. She treats patients with a variety of conditions, including osteoporosis, diabetes mellitus, and thyroid disease.

Liwei Huang, Graduated from the Sun Yat-sen University of Medical Science. After completing internal medicine and nephrology fellowship training at the Peking Union Medical College Hospital she moved to the United States to work as a postdoctoral fellow at the University of Illinois at Chicago. She then completed her internal medical residency training at the University of Tennessee and nephrology fellowship training at the University of Pennsylvania. She served as an instructor at the Department of Medicine at the University of Pennsylvania from 2012 to 2013.

She joined the nephrology division of the Eastern Virginia Medical School in 2013 as an assistant professor. Dr Huang is board certified by the American Board of Internal Medicine in Internal Medicine and subspecialty in Nephrology. Her professional memberships include American Society of Nephrology and International Society of Nephrology.

In clinical practice she focuses on the overlap of diabetes and high blood pressure and concurrent kidney disease, end-stage renal disease, and acute hospital nephrology care.

Romesh Khardori, MD, obtained his medical degree from the All-India Institute of Medical Sciences, New Delhi (India), and completed his postdoctoral fellowship in Endocrinology and Metabolism at Oregon Health Sciences Center, Portland, Oregon. This was followed by fellowship in Medicine, Diabetes, and Endocrinology at Joslin Diabetes Center, New England Deaconess, Beth Israel Hospital, Harvard Medical School, Boston, MA. Professor Khardori is currently serving as Professor of Endocrinology and Metabolism at Eastern Virginia Medical School in Norfolk, VA. Prior to this position, he was Professor and Director of the Division of Endocrinology, Metabolism and Molecular Medicine at Southern Illinois University School of Medicine in Springfield, Illinois.

Professor Khardori is ABIM board certified in Endocrinology, Diabetes, and Metabolism and has over 250+ publications. He serves as Associate Editor for *Frontiers in Endocrinology* and *Diabetes*, as well as Chief Editor of Endocrinology-Diabetes and Endocrine Emergencies for Medscape/WebMD.

Daisuke Koya, MD, PhD is the Department Chief of Metabolism and Endocrinology for Kanazawa Medical University hospital and a Chief and Professor of Diabetology and Endocrinology at Kanazawa Medical University. He received his Ph.D. degree from Shiga University of Medical Science and completed his postdoctoral training in Joslin Diabetes Center at the Harvard Medical University. His main research activities involve the study of protein kinase C, sirtuin, and autophagy in obesity, diabetes, and aging-related kidney disease.

Iyad Mansour, MD, completed his medical school training at Misr University of Science and Technology, Egypt, and received internal medicine training at The Islamic Hospital in Amman, Jordan. He then worked at King Hussain Cancer Center in Jordan as a hospitalist in a bone marrow transplant unit. Dr. Mansour moved to the United States in 2013 and started his training in internal medicine at the University of Arizona, where he is a third-year internal medicine resident and is embarking on a nephrology fellowship. In 2014, Dr. Mansour was selected by the University of Arizona as an outstanding nephrology resident. His research interests include glomerulonephritis, electrolyte disturbance, and diabetic kidney disease.

Mark E. Molitch, MD, is the Martha Leland Sherwin Professor of Endocrinology at Northwestern University Feinberg School of Medicine in Chicago, Illinois. He trained in internal medicine at the Hospital of the University of Pennsylvania and in endocrinology at UCLA-Harbor General Hospital. He performs clinical research and treats patients with a variety of endocrine conditions, including diabetes mellitus and pituitary disease.

Friedrich C. Prischl, MD, is an Associate Professor of Medicine at the Klinikum Wels-Grieskirchen, in Wels, Austria. He trained in internal medicine at the Department of Medicine, Vienna University Medical School, and is board certified in internal medicine, nephrology, hematology and oncology, and geriatric medicine. He has published over 50 manuscripts in peer-reviewed journals (as of April 2016), and more than 60 other papers (such as book chapters, reviews for national journals).

Bijin Thajudeen, MD, FACP, FASN, was born in October of 1976, in Kerala, India. He did his medical school training at the prestigious University of Kerala Medical College, Thiruvananthapuram, India. He trained in internal medicine and nephrology at the University of Arizona, Tucson, Arizona, USA. Dr Thajudeen's practice specializes in the care of patients with diabetes-related kidney diseases. His research interests include diabetic nephropathy, acute kidney injury, critical care nephrology, and the use of telemedicine in the care of patients. Dr Thajudeen is currently a clinical Assistant Professor of Nephrology at the UA Division of Nephrology and a staff member at Banner – University Medical Center Tucson. He is a fellow of the American College of Physicians and American Society of Nephrologists. Dr Thajudeen is board certified in internal medicine and nephrology. He serves as an editorial board member and reviewer for several journals. He has numerous peer-reviewed publications in national and international journals.

Contents

Contributors

Liwei Huang Division of Nephrology, Eastern Virginia Medical School, Norfolk, VA, USA

Colleen Majewski Section of Endocrinology, University of Chicago Medicine, Chicago, IL, USA

Iyad Mansour Department of Medicine, University of Arizona College of Medicine, Tucson, AZ, USA

Chapter 1
Overview of Diabetic Nephropathy

Iyad Mansour and Bijin Thajudeen

1.1 Introduction

Diabetes mellitus (DM) is an increasing global public health problem characterized by β-cell dysfunction and insulin resistance. The prevalence of DM is increasing worldwide due to aging populations, physical inactivity, obesity, rapid urbanization, and changing lifestyle and food consumption patterns [1]. According to the International Diabetes Federation, the number of people with diabetes worldwide is projected to increase from 382 million in 2013 to 592 million by 2035 [2]. Diabetic nephropathy (DN), also known as diabetic kidney disease (DKD), is one of the most important long-term complications of diabetes and the most common cause of end-stage renal disease (ESRD) worldwide. DKD occurs in type 1 and type 2 diabetes mellitus and other secondary forms of diabetes and is defined as structural and functional renal damage manifested as clinically detected albuminuria in the presence of normal or abnormal glomerular filtration rate (GFR). It is also regarded as a characteristic microvascular complication of diabetes that is related to the duration of diabetes and involves complex interactions between environmental factors and genetic determinants.

DKD develops over the initial 10–15 years of disease onset in type 1 diabetes, whereas the onset is not clearly defined in type 2 due to the late diagnosis of diabetes in some patients.

G.L. Bakris et al., *Managing Diabetic Nephropathies in Clinical Practice*, DOI 10.1007/978-3-319-08873-0_1,
© Springer International Publishing Switzerland 2017

It is also known that the longer life expectancy of the diabetic population and improved treatment and disease management have significant influence on the incidence and prevalence of DKD [3]. Patients with DKD also account for one-third of patients demanding renal transplantation. All these factors impart a huge burden on the health-care costs and resources. For example, in the United States, Medicare expenditure on treating ESRD is approximately US $33 billion (as of 2010), which accounts for 8–9 % of the total annual health-care budget. In 2009, overall Medicare expenditure for people with DKD accounted for US $18 billion, and it continues to increase [4]. Hence, surveillance, prevention, and control of DM, DKD, and related complications are becoming increasingly important.

1.2   Diagnosis of Diabetic Kidney Disease

The diagnosis of DKD is usually based on clinical information and patient health history. Renal biopsy is not commonly performed in patients with diabetes, and is usually reserved for those with unexplained rapid deterioration of renal function or suspected secondary renal disease. Factors which favor DKD diagnosis (especially in type 1) include a long history of diabetes, history of proteinuria preceding impairment in renal function, presence of diabetic retinopathy, and presence of large kidneys or relatively preserved kidneys on ultrasound [5, 6].

In terms of histopathology, DKD is characterized by hypertrophy and expansion in the glomerular mesangium, thickening of glomerular basement membrane, reduction in podocyte number, podocyte dysfunction, and accumulation of extracellular matrix (ECM) proteins resulting from an imbalance in synthesis and degradation [7–10]. Morphological changes are also seen in the tubulo-interstitium and intrarenal vasculature. Tubulo-interstitium changes include fibrosis, while vascular changes include arteriolar thickening and hyalinization. The earliest marker of renal involvement in DKD is proteinuria. But at the same time, it should also be noted that kidneys might have already been significantly damaged by the time proteinuria appears, and, hence, preventative action against developing ESRD may be too late at this stage [11, 12].

1.3   Epidemiology

More than 150 million people are affected with DKD worldwide. DKD affects about 30 % of patients with type 1 diabetes and 25–40 % of the patients with type 2 diabetes. However, the prevalence of DKD in existing or incident ESRD patients varies in different parts of the world. Table 1.1 shows a sam-

TABLE 1.1 Prevalence of diabetes kidney disease (DKD) in patients with existing or incident end-stage renal disease (ESRD)

Country [reference]	Percentage of DKD patients (%)
France [13]	56
Japan [14]	45
United States [15]	45
Korea [16]	44.9
Taiwan [15]	44.5
Australia/New Zealand [17]	35
United Kingdom [17]	25.3
Saudi Arabia [18]	20
Italy [19]	20
Norway [19]	10–15
China [20]	15
Finland [21]	7.8 (type 1)
Sweden [22]	3.3 (type 1)

ple of DKD-related ESRD in a cross section of countries to illustrate this variation [13–22].

The global prevalence of proteinuria in DKD also varies based on geographical location. The global prevalence of micro- and macroalbuminuria is estimated at 39 % and 10 %, respectively, based on the study findings of Parving et al. [23]. The National Health and Nutrition Examination Survey (NHANES III) also reported a prevalence of 35 % (microalbuminuria) and 6 % (macroalbuminuria) in patients with T2DM aged ≥40 years [24]. In another study, this was reported to be 43 % and 12 %, respectively, in a Japanese population [23]. According to the European Diabetes (EURODIAB) Prospective Complications Study Group, in patients with T1DM, the incidence of microalbuminuria was 12.6 % (over 7.3 years) [25]. This prevalence was further estimated at 33 % in an 18-year follow-up study in Denmark [26]. In the United Kingdom Prospective Diabetes Study (UKPDS), proteinuria occurred in 15–40 % of patients with T1DM, with a peak incidence after around 15–20 years after diabetes diagnosis. But in patients with T2DM, the prevalence ranged from 5 to 20 % [27]. In the Diabetes Control and Complications Trial (DCCT), which analyzed patients with estimated GFR <60 mL/min, the prevalence of normoalbuminuria, microalbuminuria, and macroalbuminuria was 24 %, 16 %, and 61 %, respectively [28].

Certain ethnic groups seem to be at greater risk of developing nephropathy. For example, in the United States, DKD is more prevalent among African-Americans, Asians, and Native Americans than Caucasians [29].

1.3.1   Staging of Diabetic Kidney Disease

Conventionally, DKD is divided into five stages:

- *Stage 1*: reversible glomerular hyperfiltration
- *Stage 2*: normal GFR and normoalbuminuria

- *Stage 3*: microalbuminuria and normal GFR (approximately 5–10 years after diagnosis of DM)
- *Stage 4*: presence of proteinuria; may reach nephrotic levels (usually 10-15 years of disease)
- *Stage 5*: chronic kidney disease which leads to terminal kidney disease (usual GFR slope <10 mL/min/year) [30]

In terms of functionality, DKD can also be divided into five distinct stages [31, 32]:

- *Stage 1*: Hyperfunction and hypertrophy. Changes are usually found at diagnosis in type 1 diabetes. Exaggerated urinary albumin excretion is present and can be aggravated during physical exercise. At this stage, changes are partially reversible by insulin treatment.
- *Stage 2*: Morphologic lesions without signs of clinical disease and increased GFR. Albumin excretion can be normal during this phase. Poor glycemic control and lack of physical exercise can unmask albuminuria. These lesions often develop silently over many years.
- *Stage 3*: Incipient DN, forerunner of overt DN. It is characterized by abnormally elevated urinary albumin excretion (measured by radioimmunoassay). There is a progressive rise in albuminuria during this phase, starting from microalbuminuria (30–300 mg albumin/day [24 h]) to macroalbuminuria (>300 mg/day). Albumin excretion is higher in patients with increased blood pressure (BP). GFR can still be supernormal during the phase.
- *Stage 4*: Overt DN. It is characterized by persistent proteinuria (>0.5 g/day) and a reduction in GFR.
- *Stage 5*: ESRD with uremia due to DKD.

Based on the histopathological findings, DKD can be classified as shown in Table 1.2 [33]. Additionally, based on the presence of interstitial and vascular lesions, a scoring system has been put forth (Table 1.3) [33]. According to this system, interstitial lesions can be divided into those having interstitial

TABLE 1.2 Classification of diabetic kidney disease based on histopathology

Class	Description
I	Thickening of glomerular basement membrane
II	Mesangial expansion It can be mild (IIa) or severe (IIb).
III	Nodular sclerosis (Kimmelstiel–Wilson lesions)
IV	Advanced diabetic glomerulosclerosis[a]

Adapted with permission from Tervaert et al. [33] ©American Society of Nephropathy.

[a]Where more than 50 % global glomerulosclerosis with other clinical or pathologic evidence that sclerosis is attributable to diabetic nephropathy

fibrosis and tubular atrophy (IFTA) and those having interstitial inflammation. Based on the percentage of IFTA, a score of 0–3 is given, and based on the location of infiltration, a score of 0–2 is given. For vascular lesions, arteriolar hyalinosis, involvement of large vessels, and arteriosclerosis are taken into consideration. Depending on the extent of arteriolar hyalinosis, a score of 0–2 is given. Arteriosclerosis is given a score of 0–2, depending on the extent of intimal thickening [33].

1.3.2   The Natural History of Diabetic Kidney Disease

A natural history of DKD was first described in the 1970s by Danish physicians [32]. It was characterized by a long silent period without overt clinical signs and symptoms of nephropathy and progression through various stages, starting from hyperfiltration, microalbuminuria, macroalbuminuria, and overt renal failure to ESRD. Microalbuminuria (30–300 mg/day of albumin in urine) is a sign of early DKD, whereas macroalbuminuria (>300 mg/day) represents DKD progression.

However, this 'classical' natural evolution of urinary albumin excretion and change in GFR is not present in many

TABLE 1.3 Scoring system for diabetic kidney disease based on interstitial and vascular lesions

Lesion	Criteria	Score
Interstitial lesions		
IFTA	No IFTA	0
	<25 %	1
	25–50 %	2
	>50 %	3
Interstitial inflammation	Absent	0
	Infiltration in areas of IFTA	1
	Infiltration in areas without IFTA	2
Vascular lesions		
Arteriolar hyalinosis	Absent	0
	At least one area of arteriolar hyalinosis	1
	More than one area of arteriolar hyalinosis	2
Presence of large vessels	–	Yes/No
Arteriosclerosis	No intimal thickening	0
	Intimal thickening less than thickness of media	1
	Intimal thickening greater than thickness of media	2

IFTA, interstitial fibrosis and tubular atrophy. Reproduced with permission from Tervaert et al. [33] ©American Society of Nephropathy.

patients with diabetes, especially those with type 2 diabetes [34]. These patients can have reduction or disappearance of proteinuria over time or can develop even overt renal disease in the absence of proteinuria [30, 35]. This heterogeneous presentation can be influenced by factors such as hypertensive, atherosclerotic, and ischemic nephropathy, rather than a typical heavily proteinuric nephropathy [36]. They can also develop other glomerular diseases, including immunoglobulin A (IgA) nephropathy, membranous nephropathy, or lupus nephritis, among other conditions.

The heterogeneity in presentation has been demonstrated in observational studies. In the Wisconsin Epidemiologic Study of Diabetic Retinopathy (WESDR) of patients with T2DM, 45.2 % of participants developed albuminuria, and 29 % developed renal impairment over a 15-year follow-up period [37]. Of those patients who developed renal impairment, 61 % did not have albuminuria beforehand, and 39 % never developed albuminuria during the study. Of the patients that developed albuminuria, only 24 % subsequently developed renal impairment during the study. A significant degree of discordance between development of albuminuria and renal impairment is apparent [37]. These data, thus, do not support the classical paradigm of albuminuria always preceding renal impairment in the progression of DKD. These findings also suggest that microalbuminuria alone may not provide optimal identification of patients with T2DM at higher risk of renal impairment.

A number of risk factors other than proteinuria have been associated with onset and progression of DKD (Fig. 1.1) [6, 20, 23, 38–48]. Certain groups (e.g., Italian, Brazilian, Indian, Caucasian American, Japanese, Turkish, Pima, and African-American) have higher risk for progression of DKD compared to others ethnicities. Factors that might be playing a role for this ethnic variation include differences in access to health care, prevalence of modifiable lifestyle risk factors, and an inherited predisposition to DKD [25, 27, 49]. Hypertension is present in majority of patients with DKD, and it plays an important role in the progression of DKD [25]. Effective blood pressure control is associated with reduced incidence of albuminuria and the development of ESRD [50]. A 'non-dipping' of nocturnal blood pressure in normo-albuminuric patients with T1DM was found

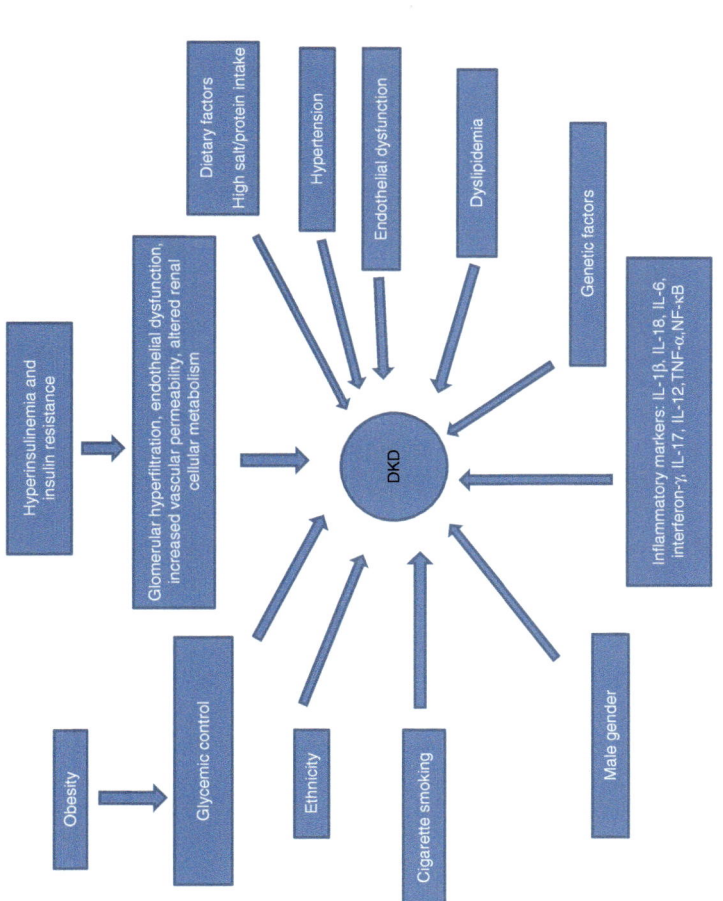

FIGURE 1.1 Risk factors associated with onset and progression of diabetic kidney disease (DKD)

to predict microalbuminuria, whereas in T2DM patients, an abnormal circadian BP profile is strongly correlated with the presence of albuminuria. A non-dipping BP pattern is also associated with overt proteinuria and higher morbidity and mortality in patients with DM [51]. In addition, a number of minor factors may also play a role. For example, physical-inherited factors including short stature, intrauterine growth retardation, and low birth weight may make patients with diabetes more susceptible to DKD [52].

Patients with DKD have a predisposition to develop renal injury from various sources, which include contrast-induced injury, volume depletion, and the use of nonsteroidal anti-inflammatory drugs [53].

Pregnancy is also associated with a worsening of microvascular or macrovascular disease, including DKD [54, 55]. Advanced glycation end products, high plasma asymmetric dimethylarginine, high serum fibroblast growth factor 23 (FGF-23), hyperuricemia, hyperphosphatemia, suboptimal vitamin D levels, angiotensinogen, angiotensin receptor II, aldolase, apolipoprotein E, intracellular adhesion molecules, nitric oxide synthase, and vascular endothelial growth factors are common biochemical factors that have been found to be associated with higher risk of DKD progression [26, 43, 48, 56–58].

Although there are many factors that can influence the development and progression of DKD, one single factor is insufficient to predict the onset of the disease. Genetic factors might also play a role. The role of genetic predisposition is evidenced by the discovery of a familial association for the development of DKD in siblings of diabetic probands, causing a threefold increase in DKD risk [59]. Genetic studies have found a familial aggregation of DKD (albuminuria, overt nephropathy, and ESRD) in both type 1 and type 2 diabetes, which varies depending on the patient's ethic background [15, 60].

Based on candidate gene approaches and genome-wide linkage analyses, several candidate genes have been found to have a potential impact on specific aspects of DKD. For example, in Asian populations, a single nucleotide polymorphism in the *ACACB* gene is strongly associated with the development of albuminuria [61]. In Chinese patients with type 2 diabetes, polymorphisms in the protein kinase C-β1 (*PKCB1*) gene have been associated with increased risk of ESRD [62]. A meta-analysis of 18 studies showed a relationship between the Pro12Ala polymorphism in the human peroxisome proliferator-activated receptor gamma (*PPARG*) gene and improved insulin sensitivity, decreased risk of type 2 diabetes, and lower levels of albuminuria and diabetic nephroprathy in Caucasians (no similar association was observed in Asian populations) [63]. Other genes that have been found to have an association with predisposition to DKD [64–66] include:

- Sirtuin 1 (*SIRT1*)
- Angiotensin-converting enzyme (*ACE*)
- Myosin, heavy chain 9, non-muscle (*MYH9*)
- Fatty acid-binding protein 2, instrinal (*FABP2*)
- Ectonucleotide pyrophosphatase/phosphodiesterase 1 (*ENPP1*)
- FERM domain containing 3 (*FRMD3*)
- Cysteinyl-tRNA synthetase (*CARS*)
- Serine carboxypeptidase vitellogenic-like (*CPVL*)
- Glucose transporter 1 (GLUT1) on the solute carrier family 2, facilitated glucose transporter member 1 (*SLC2A1*) gene

These genetic factors have been linked to development of ESRD, microalbuminuria, and insulin resistance [52, 59].

1.4   Glomerular Filtration Rate Estimation

Assessment of renal function is an essential tool for nephrologists and diabetologists, and thus, an estimation of GFR (eGRF) is crucial at each stage of DKD. In fact, renal hyperfiltration and rapid GFR decline are considered stronger predictors of nephropathy progression in type 1 diabetes than presence of albuminuria [67]. The annual eGFR loss in patients with DKD is >3 mL/min/1.73 m^2 or 3.3 % per year.

Various methods such as using a creatinine- or cystatin (Cys C)-based equation can be used for estimating GFR. Creatinine-based GFR estimates are influenced by confounders, including filtration fraction (FF = GFR/effective renal plasma flow), muscle mass, and renal tubular secretion. This can impact the use of creatinine, especially in the presence of hyperfiltration. The

Modification of Diet in Renal Disease (MDRD) study equation is one of the most widely used creatinine-based methods to calculate eGFR and has been validated in Caucasian and African-American patients over 18 years of age [68]. However, the use of the MDRD study equation may cause an underestimated GFR result when eGFR is >60 mL/min/1.73 m^2 and, in some patients, if it is between 45 and 60 mL/min/1.73 m^2. Reasons for this underestimation include disparity in the calibration of serum creatinine, measurement error, variability in the distribution of GFR, as well as clinical characteristics which in turn affect the accuracy of MDRD study equation [69]. In spite of these limitations, the MDRD study equation is recommended for screening by the National Kidney Foundation (NKF). However, the Chronic Kidney Disease-Epidemiology Collaboration (CKD-EPI) creatinine equation is recommended by some national bodies (e.g., National Institute of Clinical Health and Excellence [NICE] in the United Kingdom) and should also be considered [70].

GFR estimation using Cys C appears to predict the outcomes in T1DM more accurately than creatinine-based equations, especially with regard to progression to ESRD and mortality. It can estimate GFR more accurately than creatinine-based measurements in patients with type 1 diabetes with normal renal function. A reduction in eGFR using Cys C can predict cardiovascular complications and mortality and is also thought to be superior in terms of detecting acute changes in eGFR induced by hyperglycemia [4, 64, 71]. However, there are contradicting reports of the use of Cys C in patients with diabetes. Some studies have shown no advantage of Cys C-based equations in GFR over creatinine-based equation (e.g., MDRD) in patients with either type 1 or type 2 diabetes [72, 73]. It is affected by a number of factors similar to creatinine-based equations, and hence there is a need to standardize Cys C calibration to enable the more widespread use of eGFR-estimating equations using Cys C [67]. GFR estimation incorporating both creatinine- and Cys C-based equations might give a better correlation with true GFR levels.

There are other major challenges in the measurement of GFR which are specific to DM. Several factors like hyperglycemia, excessive intake of caffeine, protein load, exercise, and certain medications (e.g., diuretics, antibiotics) can interfere with the measurement of eGFR. Hyperglycemia (especially blood glucose concentrations >300 mg/dL) can cause an over-estimate of the GFR, leading to an increase of up to 20 mL/min/1.73 m^2 [4].

Because of the limitations of using creatinine or Cys C in estimating GFR and the fact that previous 'gold standard' measurements such as iothalamate or inulin clearance are costly and time consuming, newer methods are being developed to accurately measure GFR in patients with DM. One such method is measuring iohexol clearance [71]. Investigators are also looking at biomarkers which can predict development of DKD. β-trace protein and $β_2$-microglobulin levels are two such markers which have been found to be associated with increased risk of incident ESRD. Both of these biomarkers are filtered by the kidneys and tend to accumulate in patients with DKD. These biomarkers also have associations with cardiovascular disease, and all-cause mortality [74].

1.5   Screening for Diabetic Kidney Disease

Estimation of albumin excretion rate and GFR are the two laboratory parameters used for the screening of DKD, which varies based on the type of diabetes [75]. For type 1, screening is recommended as soon as the diagnosis is made, whereas screening for type 2 diabetes is recommended 5 years after the initial diagnosis. In the absence of microalbuminuria, screening must be repeated annually for both types. Screening methods recommended by the American Diabetes Association (ADA) include measurement of albumin in a spot urine sample collected either as the first urine in the morning or at random. The results can be expressed as urinary albumin concentration (mg/L) or as urinary albumin-to-creatinine ratio (mg/g). A cutoff value of 17 mg/L in a random urine specimen had a sensitivity of 100 % and a specificity of 80 % for the diagnosis of microalbuminuria. The test should be confirmed by repeated positive results in 2 of 3 samples collected over a period of 3- to 6-month period. A 24-hour or timed urine collection is not routinely recommended because it is cumbersome and prone to errors related to collecting samples or recording of time. It is also recommended to avoid screening in the presence of conditions which can increase urinary albumin excretion such as urinary tract infection, hematuria, acute febrile illness, vigorous exercise, short-term pronounced hyperglycemia, uncontrolled hypertension, and heart failure [4, 27].

Alternate options for measurement of albuminuria include a qualitative and semiquantitative simple dipstick measurement (e.g., Micral Test II). Because dipstick methods are not sensitive enough to detect small amounts of albuminuria, a follow-up quantitative analysis should also be performed. Immunoreactive and immunounreactive forms of liquid chromatography for measuring albumin may allow early detection of incipient DKD.

Because albuminuria is not present in all patients with DKD, measurement of eGFR is also important in the screening of DN. The ADA, NKF, and International Society of Nephrology recommend measuring eGFR annually to identify and monitor DKD [4].

1.6   Diabetic Kidney Disease and Mortality

Comorbid DM and DKD are associated with high cardiovascular morbidity and mortality. The risk of cardiovascular disease is disproportionately higher in patients with DKD than patients with DM who do not have kidney disease [76]. The incident dialysis rate might even be higher after adjusting for patients dying from cardiovascular disease before reaching ESRD stage [19]. The United States Renal Data System (USRDS) data shows that elderly patients with a triad of DM, chronic kidney disease (CKD), and heart failure have a five-fold higher chance of death than progression to CKD and ESRD [36]. The 5-year survival rate for diabetic patients with ESRD is estimated at 20 %, likely because they tend to have higher comorbidity rates and worse outcomes than nondiabetic patients on hemodialysis [10]. This is higher than the mortality rate for many solid cancers (including prostate, breast, or renal cell cancer).

Patients with diabetes also have high prevalence of protein–energy malnutrition, which can also predispose patients with ESRD to a higher likelihood of mortality, especially those undergoing peritoneal dialysis. But at the same time, overall mortality has decreased considerably in the last 30–40 years, mainly due to the aggressive hypertension management, use of renoprotective agents blocking renin–angiotensin system, and newer treatment for improving glycemic control, especially in type 1 diabetes [12].

References

1. Al-Rubeaan K, Youssef AM, Subhani SN, Ahmad NA, Al-Sharqawi AH, Al-Mutlag HM, et al. Diabetic nephropathy and its risk factors in a society with a type 2 diabetes epidemic: a Saudi National Diabetes Registry-based study. PLoS One. 2014;9:e88956.
2. Ding Y, Choi ME. Autophagy in diabetic nephropathy. J Endocrinol. 2015;224:R15–30.
3. Arslan D, Merdin A, Tural D, Temizel M, Akin O, Güdüz S, Tatlı AM, et al. The effect of autoimmunity on the development time of microvascular complications in patients with type 1 diabetes mellitus. Med Sci Monit. 2014;20:1176–9.
4. Bjornstad P, Cherney DZ, Maahs DM. Update on estimation of kidney function in diabetic kidney disease. Curr Diab Rep. 2015;15:57.
5. Park CW. Diabetic kidney disease: from epidemiology to clinical perspectives. Diabetes Metab J. 2014;38:252–60.
6. Lampropoulou IT, Stangou M, Papagianni A, Didangelos T, Iliadis F, Efstratiadis G. TNF-α and microalbuminuria in patients with type 2 diabetes mellitus. J Diabetes Res. 2014;2014:394206.
7. Al-Malki AL. Assessment of urinary osteopontin in association with podocyte for early predication of nephropathy in diabetic patients. Dis Markers. 2014;2014:493736.
8. Brosius FC, Coward RJ. Podocytes, signaling pathways, and vascular factors in diabetic kidney disease. Adv Chronic Kidney Dis. 2014;21:304–10.
9. Coward R, Fornoni A. Insulin signaling: implications for podocyte biology in diabetic kidney disease. Curr Opin Nephrol Hypertens. 2015;24:104–10.
10. Xu X, Xiao L, Xiao P, Yang S, Chen G, Liu F, et al. A glimpse of matrix metalloproteinases in diabetic nephropathy. Curr Med Chem. 2014;21:3244–60.

11. Higgins GC, Coughlan MT. Mitochondrial dysfunction and mitophagy: the beginning and end to diabetic nephropathy? Br J Pharmacol. 2014;171:1917–42.
12. Siwy J, Schanstra JP, Argiles A, Bakker SJ, Beige J, Boucek P, et al. Multicentre prospective validation of a urinary peptidome-based classifier for the diagnosis of type 2 diabetic nephropathy. Nephrol Dial Transplant. 2014;29:1563–70.
13. Couchoud C, Villar E. End-stage renal disease epidemic in diabetics: is there light at the end of the tunnel? Nephrol Dial Transplant. 2013;28:1073–76.
14. Katayama S, Moriya T, Tanaka S, Tanaka S, Yajima Y, Sone H, et al. Low transition rate from normo- and low microalbuminuria to proteinuria in Japanese type 2 diabetic individuals: the Japan Diabetes Complications Study (JDCS). Diabetologia. 2011;54:1025–31.
15. Liao LN, Chen CC, Wu FY, Lin CC, Hsiao JH, Chang CT, et al. Identified single-nucleotide polymorphisms and haplotypes at 16q22.1 increase diabetic nephropathy risk in Han Chinese population. BMC Genet. 2014;15:113.
16. Chung SH, Han DC, Noh H, Jeon JS, Kwon SH, Lindholm B, et al. Risk factors for mortality in diabetic peritoneal dialysis patients. Nephrol Dial Transplant. 2010;25:3742–8.
17. Grace BS, Clayton P, McDonald SP. Increases in renal replacement therapy in Australia and New Zealand: understanding trends in diabetic nephropathy. Nephrology (Carlton). 2012;17:76–84.
18. Alwakeel JS, Isnani AC, Alsuwaida A, Alharbi A, Shaffi SA, Almohaya S, et al. Factors affecting the progression of diabetic nephropathy and its complications: a single-center experience in Saudi Arabia. Ann Saudi Med. 2011;31:236–42.
19. Fabbian F, De Giorgi A, Monesi M, Pala M, Tiseo R, Misurati E, et al. All-cause mortality and estimated renal function in type 2 diabetes mellitus outpatients: Is there a relationship with the equation used? Diab Vasc Dis Res. 2015;12:46–52.
20. Magee GM, Hunter SJ, Cardwell CR, Savage G, Kee F, Murphy MC, et al. Identifying additional patients with diabetic nephropathy using the UK primary care initiative. Diabet Med. 2010;27:1372–8.
21. Finne P, Reunanen A, Stenman S, Groop PH, Grönhagen-Riska C. Incidence of end-stage renal disease in patients with type 1 diabetes. JAMA. 2005;294:1782–7.
22. Afghahi H, Cederholm J, Eliasson B, Zethelius B, Gudbjörnsdottir S, Hadimeri H, et al. Risk factors for the development of albu-

minuria and renal impairment in type 2 diabetes – the Swedish National Diabetes Register (NDR). Nephrol Dial Transplant. 2011;26:1236–43.

23. Kawabata N, Kawamura T, Utsunomiya K, Kusano E. High salt intake is associated with renal involvement in Japanese patients with type 2 diabetes mellitus. Intern Med. 2015;54:311–7.

24. Coresh J, Selvin E, Stevens LA, Manzi J, Kusek JW, Eggers P, et al. Prevalence of chronic kidney disease in the United States. JAMA. 2007;298:2038–47.

25. Van Buren PN, Toto R. Hypertension in diabetic nephropathy: epidemiology, mechanisms, and management. Adv Chronic Kidney Dis. 2011;18:28–41.

26. Hovind P, Tarnow L, Rossing P, Jensen BR, Graae M, Torp I, et al. Predictors for the development of microalbuminuria and macroalbuminuria in patients with type 1 diabetes: inception cohort study. BMJ. 2004;328:1105.

27. Gross JL, de Azevedo MJ, Silveiro SP, Canani LH, Caramori ML, Zelmanovitz T. Diabetic nephropathy: diagnosis, prevention, and treatment. Diabetes Care. 2005;28:164–76.

28. Molitch ME, Steffes M, Sun W, Rutledge B, Cleary P, de Boer IH, et al. Development and progression of renal insufficiency with and without albuminuria in adults with type 1 diabetes in the diabetes control and complications trial and the epidemiology of diabetes interventions and complications study. Diabetes Care. 2010;33:1536–43.

29. Burrows NR, Cho P, McKeever Bullard K, Narva AS, Eggers PW. Survival on dialysis among American Indians and Alaska Natives with diabetes in the United States, 1995-2010. Am J Public Health. 2014;104 Suppl 3:S490–5.

30. Halimi JM. The emerging concept of chronic kidney disease without clinical proteinuria in diabetic patients. Diabetes Metab. 2012;38:291–7.

31. Haneda M, Utsunomiya K, Koya D, Babazono T, Moriya T, Makino H, et al. A new classification of diabetic nephropathy 2014: a report from Joint Committee on Diabetic Nephropathy. J Diabetes Investig. 2015;6:242–6.

32. Mogensen CE, Christensen CK, Vittinghus E. The stages in diabetic renal disease. With emphasis on the stage of incipient diabetic nephropathy. Diabetes. 1983;32 Suppl 2:64–78.

33. Tervaert TW, Mooyaart AL, Amann K, Cohen AK, Cook HT, Drachenberg CB, et al. Pathologic classification of diabetic nephropathy. J Am Soc Nephrol. 2010;21:556–3.

34. MacIsaac RJ, Tsalamandris C, Panagiotopoulos S, Smith TJ, McNeil KJ, Jerums G. Nonalbuminuric renal insufficiency in type 2 diabetes. Diabetes Care. 2004;27:195–200.
35. Rigalleau V, Lasseur C, Raffaitin C, Cohen AH, Cook HT, Drachenberg CB, et al. Normoalbuminuric renal-insufficient diabetic patients: a lower-risk group. Diabetes Care. 2007;30:2034–9.
36. Altemtam N, Russell J, El Nahas M. A study of the natural history of diabetic kidney disease (DKD). Nephrol Dial Transplant. 2012;27:1847–54.
37. Retnakaran R, Cull CA, Thorne KI, Adler AI, Holman RR, Group US. Risk factors for renal dysfunction in type 2 diabetes: UK Prospective Diabetes Study 74. Diabetes. 2006;55:1832–9.
38. De Cosmo S, Menzaghi C, Prudente S, Trischitta V. Role of insulin resistance in kidney dysfunction: insights into the mechanism and epidemiological evidence. Nephrol Dial Transplant. 2013;28:29–36.
39. Downs CA, Faulkner MS. Toxic stress, inflammation and symptomatology of chronic complications in diabetes. World J Diabetes. 2015;6:554–65.
40. Hua P, Feng W, Ji S, Raij L, Jaimes EA. Nicotine worsens the severity of nephropathy in diabetic mice: implications for the progression of kidney disease in smokers. Am J Physiol Renal Physiol. 2010;299:F732–9.
41. Huang Y, Liu Y, Li L, Su B, Yang L, Fan W, et al. Involvement of inflammation-related miR-155 and miR-146a in diabetic nephropathy: implications for glomerular endothelial injury. BMC Nephrol. 2014;15:142.
42. Liu F, Fu P. Management of glycemia in diabetic patients with diabetic kidney disease. Chin Med J (Engl). 2014;127:1170–6.
43. Maric C, Forsblom C, Thorn L, Wadén J, Groop PH, Group FS. Association between testosterone, estradiol and sex hormone binding globulin levels in men with type 1 diabetes with nephropathy. Steroids. 2010;75:772–8.
44. Ritz E, Orth SR. Nephropathy in patients with type 2 diabetes mellitus. N Engl J Med. 1999;341:1127–33.
45. Takahashi T, Harris RC. Role of endothelial nitric oxide synthase in diabetic nephropathy: lessons from diabetic eNOS knockout mice. J Diabetes Res. 2014;2014:590541.
46. Whitham D. Nutrition for the prevention and treatment of chronic kidney disease in diabetes. Can J Diabetes. 2014;38:344–8.
47. Ngarmukos C, Bunnag P, Kosachunhanun N, Krittiyawong S, Leelawatana R, Prathipanawatr T, et al. Thailand diabetes registry

project: prevalence, characteristics and treatment of patients with diabetic nephropathy. J Med Assoc Thai. 2006;89:S37–42.

48. Gao C, Huang W, Kanasaki K, Xu Y. The role of ubiquitination and sumoylation in diabetic nephropathy. Biomed Res Int. 2014;2014:160692.

49. Thameem F, Kawalit IA, Adler SG, Abboud HE. Susceptibility gene search for nephropathy and related traits in Mexican-Americans. Mol Biol Rep. 2013;40:5769–79.

50. Hotu C, Bagg W, Collins J, Harwood L, Whalley G, Doughty R, et al. A community-based model of care improves blood pressure control and delays progression of proteinuria, left ventricular hypertrophy and diastolic dysfunction in Maori and Pacific patients with type 2 diabetes and chronic kidney disease: a randomized controlled trial. Nephrol Dial Transplant. 2010;25:3260–6.

51. Jindal A, Garcia-Touza M, Jindal N, Whaley-Connell A, Sowers JR. Diabetic kidney disease and the cardiorenal syndrome: old disease, new perspectives. Endocrinol Metab Clin North Am. 2013;42:789–808.

52. Fava S, Hattersley AT. The role of genetic susceptibility in diabetic nephropathy: evidence from family studies. Nephrol Dial Transplant. 2002;17:1543–6.

53. Calvin AD, Misra S, Pflueger A. Contrast-induced acute kidney injury and diabetic nephropathy. Nat Rev Nephrol. 2010;6:679–88.

54. Piccoli GB, Clari R, Ghiotto S, Castelluccia N, Colombi N, Mauro G, et al. Type 1 diabetes, diabetic nephropathy, and pregnancy: a systematic review and meta-study. Rev Diabet Stud. 2013;10:6–26.

55. Sandvik MK, Iversen BM, Irgens LM, Skjaerven R, Leivestad T, Søfteland E, et al. Are adverse pregnancy outcomes risk factors for development of end-stage renal disease in women with diabetes? Nephrol Dial Transplant. 2010;25:3600–7.

56. Bonakdaran S, Hami M, Shakeri MT. Hyperuricemia and albuminuria in patients with type 2 diabetes mellitus. Iran J Kidney Dis. 2011;5:21–4.

57. Mager DR, Jackson ST, Hoffmann MR, Jindal K, Senior PA. Vitamin D supplementation and bone health in adults with diabetic nephropathy: the protocol for a randomized controlled trial. BMC Endocr Disord. 2014;14:66.

58. Yilmaz MI, Sonmez A, Saglam M, Yaman H, Cayci T, Kilic S, et al. Reduced proteinuria using ramipril in diabetic CKD stage 1 decreases circulating cell death receptor activators concurrently with ADMA. A novel pathophysiological pathway? Nephrol Dial Transplant. 2010;25:3250–6.

59. Doria A. Genetics of diabetes complications. Curr Diab Rep. 2010;10:467–75.
60. McDonough CW, Palmer ND, Hicks PJ, Roh BH, An SS, Cooke JN, et al. A genome-wide association study for diabetic nephropathy genes in African Americans. Kidney Int. 2011;79:563–72.
61. Maeda S, Kobayashi MA, Araki S, Babazono T, Freedman BI, Bostrom MA, et al. A single nucleotide polymorphism within the acetyl-coenzyme A carboxylase beta gene is associated with proteinuria in patients with type 2 diabetes. PLoS Genet. 2010;6:e1000842.
62. Murea M, Ma L, Freedman BI. Genetic and environmental factors associated with type 2 diabetes and diabetic vascular complications. Rev Diabet Stud. 2012;9:6–22.
63. Zhang H, Zhu S, Chen J, Tang Y, Hu H, Mohan V, et al. Peroxisome proliferator-activated receptor γ polymorphism Pro12Ala Is associated with nephropathy in type 2 diabetes: evidence from meta-analysis of 18 studies. Diabetes Care. 2012;35:1388–93.
64. Maeda S, Koya D, Araki S, Babazono T, Umezono T, Toyoda M, et al. Association between single nucleotide polymorphisms within genes encoding sirtuin families and diabetic nephropathy in Japanese subjects with type 2 diabetes. Clin Exp Nephrol. 2011;15:381–90.
65. Pezzolesi MG, Krolewski AS. The genetic risk of kidney disease in type 2 diabetes. Med Clin North Am. 2013;97:91–107.
66. Tang ZH, Fang Z, Zhou L. Human genetics of diabetic vascular complications. J Genet. 2013;92:677–94.
67. Rigalleau V, Beauvieux MC, Gonzalez C, Raffaitin C, Lasseur C, Combe C, et al. Estimation of renal function in patients with diabetes. Diabetes Metab. 2011;37:359–66.
68. Levey AS, Stevens LA, Schmid CH, Zhang YL, Castro 3rd AF, Feldman HI, et al. A new equation to estimate glomerular filtration rate. Ann Intern Med. 2009;150:604–12.
69. Stevens LA, Coresh J, Feldman HI, Greene T, Lash JP, Nelson RG, et al. Evaluation of the modification of diet in renal disease study equation in a large diverse population. J Am Soc Nephrol. 2007;18:2749–57.
70. Chronic kidney disease in adults: assessment and management. NICE guidelines [CG182]. July 2014. www.nice.org.uk/guidance/cg182. Accessed March 11, 2016.
71. Bjornstad P, Cherney D, Maahs DM. Early diabetic nephropathy in type 1 diabetes: new insights. Curr Opin Endocrinol Diabetes Obes. 2014;21:279–86.

72. Maahs DM, Jalal D, McFann K, Rewers M, Snell-Bergeon JK. Systematic shifts in cystatin C between 2006 and 2010. Clin J Am Soc Nephrol. 2011;6:1952–5.
73. Maahs DM, Prentice N, McFann K, et al. Age and sex influence cystatin C in adolescents with and without type 1 diabetes. Diabetes Care. 2011;34:2360–2.
74. Foster MC, Inker LA, Hsu CY, et al. Filtration markers as predictors of ESRD and mortality in Southwestern American Indians with type 2 diabetes. Am J Kidney Dis. 2015;66:75–83.
75. Bjornstad P, McQueen RB, Snell-Bergeon JK, et al. Fasting blood glucose – a missing variable for GFR-estimation in type 1 diabetes? PLoS One. 2014;9:e96264.
76. Pálsson R, Patel UD. Cardiovascular complications of diabetic kidney disease. Adv Chronic Kidney Dis. 2014;21:273–80.

Chapter 2
Pathogenesis of Diabetic Nephropathy

Liwei Huang and Romesh Khardori

2.1 Introduction

Diabetic nephropathy (DN), also known as diabetic kidney disease (DKD), is a major microvascular complication of diabetes mellitus. Traditionally, it has been identified as a triad of albuminuria, hypertension, and declining renal function in patients with diabetes mellitus. Earlier estimates suggested that nephropathy affects 30 % of patients with type 1 diabetes and 20 % of patients with type 2 diabetes. Prevalence of DN is a function of the duration of diabetes. Although recent estimates suggest a decline in the incidence among those with type 1 diabetes, DN remains a serious threat to overall survival in patients with diabetes mellitus [1]. It must, however, be noted that with improved blood pressure control and renal replacement therapy, the outlook has vastly changed, with a reported 10-year survival rate of 82 % compared to 28 % in those with persistent albuminuria reported only three decades ago [2]. The utility of microalbuminuria in determining progression and prognosis is complicated by 10 % of patients with DN not having proteinuria, day-to-day variation in albumin excretion rate, regression to mean over longitudinal follow-up, and failure to demonstrate microalbuminuria as a therapeutic target in prevention of overt DN in type 1 diabetic patients subjected to intensified glycemic control.

G.L. Bakris et al., *Managing Diabetic Nephropathies in Clinical Practice*, DOI 10.1007/978-3-319-08873-0_2,
© Springer International Publishing Switzerland 2017

DN is the leading cause of chronic and end-stage renal disease (ESRD) worldwide [3]. Despite modern therapies such as hyperglycemic control, antihypertensive management, inhibition of the renin–angiotensin–aldosterone system (RAAS), and anti-inflammatory approaches, most patients continue to show progressive renal damage. This outcome suggests that the key pathogenic mechanisms involved in the induction and progression of DN remain, at least in part, active and unmodified by the presently available therapies. Understanding the pathogenesis of this disease will help identify more effective therapies to prevent the development of, or at least delay, the progression of DN.

DN is considered a disease with individual and temporal heterogeneity. The pathogenesis of DN is multifactorial, involving a complex series of molecular processes. The pathological changes of DN are composed of histopathological and functional changes which interact with each other. The progression of DN can be divided in clinical stages (Table 2.1) [4, 5]. The first clinical sign suggesting renal involvement due to diabetes is hyperfiltration characterized by an increased glomerular filtration rate (GFR) of >120 mL/min/1.73 m^2,

TABLE 2.1 Clinical stages of diabetic nephropathy

Stage	GFR (mL/min/1.73 m^2)	AER (mg/g creatinine)	Duration of diabetes (years)
1. Hyperfiltration	>120	<30	0–5
2. Microalbuminuria	Normal	30–300	5–15
3. Macroalbuminuria/ proteinuria	Normal or <90	>300	10–20
4. Progressive kidney disease	Normal or <90	>3000	15–25
5. End-stage renal disease	<15	>3000	20–10

AER albumin excretion rate, *GFR* glomerular filtration rate

followed by the onset of microalbuminuria (albumin excretion rate [AER] >30 mg/g creatinine). This, if left untreated, progresses to overt nephropathy, characterized by macroalbuminuria (AER >300 mg/24 h or >300 mg/g creatinine).

2.2   Hemodynamic Alternations

DN is characterized at its onset by glomerular hyperfiltration, which occurs in the large majority of young patients with type 1 diabetes [6]. Potential mechanisms leading to glomerular hyperfiltration include a combination of hemodynamic, vasoactive, tubular, growth-promoting, and metabolic factors (Fig. 2.1) [7].

Glomerular hyperfiltration is strongly associated with the risk of developing microalbuminuria in diabetes and

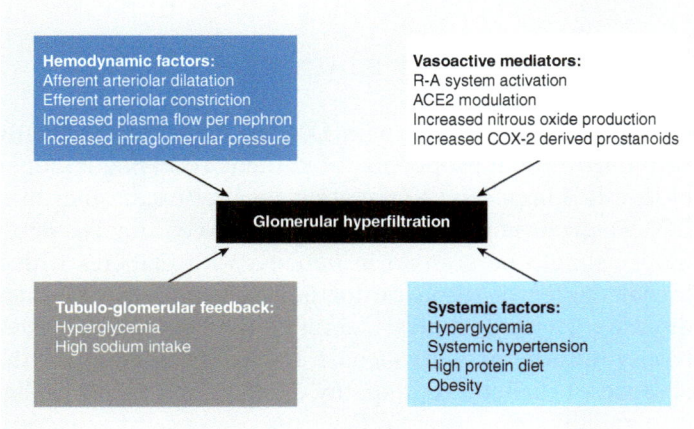

FIGURE 2.1 Glomerular hyperfiltration mechanism. Factors affecting glomerular hyperfiltration in diabetes. *ACE2* angiotensin-converting enzyme 2, *COX* cyclooxygenase, *R–A* renin–angiotensin (Reproduced with permission from Premaratne et al. [7] © Elsevier Masson)

hypertension, and it is reasonable to consider hyperfiltration as a precursor of nephropathy in these conditions [8]. A rapid GFR decline is associated with renal hyperfiltration in adults with type 1 diabetes [9], and in patients with type 2 diabetes, glomerular hyperfiltration can predict future GFR decline [10].

One problem with the diagnosis of hyperfiltration is that no generally universally accepted definition is available for this clinical entity. One reason is that GFR levels corresponding to hyperfiltration are heavily dependent on age. Thus, estimates of the prevalence of glomerular hyperfiltration in patients with type 2 diabetes vary wildly. One study showed that the prevalence of hyperfiltration was 7.4 %, but this increased to 16.6 % when age-adjusted definitions were used [11]. Moreover, recent long-term prospective surveys cast doubt on the validity of glomerular hyperfiltration being predictive of renal outcome in patients with type 1 diabetes [7].

2.3   Histopathological Changes

Currently, most patients with DN are diagnosed clinically, with only a small proportion of patients receiving a kidney biopsy. It is important to note that renal diseases other than DN can occur in patients with diabetes. Accordingly, kidney biopsy should be granted in patients with diabetes with a higher degree of suspicion for nondiabetes-related kidney disease. Atypical clinical features that promote kidney biopsy in these patients include, but are not limited to, the absence of diabetic retinopathy, rapidly increased proteinuria, rapidly decreasing GFR, or the presence of active urinary sediment (e.g., significant microscopic hematuria or pyuria).

DN is characterized by a constellation of histopathological changes including glomerular basement membrane

(GBM) thickening, mesangial expansion (in early DN), Kimmelstiel–Wilson nodules (an aggregation of mesangial cells and mesangial matrix), arterial hyalinosis, and tubu-lointerstitial changes (e.g., fibrosis and tubular atrophy in advanced DN) (Fig. 2.2) [12, 13]. Glomerular changes in DN are initiated by the direct effects of hyperglycemia, hyperlipidemia, advanced glycation end products (AGEs), and insulin-related responses (Fig. 2.3) [14].

The severity of diabetic glomerulopathy is greatly influ-enced by diabetes duration [15, 16]. Aside from mesangial matrix expansion and GBM thickening, podocyte dropout is also a critical factor for DN development. Glomerular podocyte density is the best predictor of albuminuria and progression [17, 18]. As podocytes are not readily replaced, the remaining podocytes change their size and shape to cover the portion of the GBM left 'naked' by lost podo-cytes [12, 19].

2.4 Metabolic Pathways

Several metabolically driven, glucose-dependent pathways are activated within DN. These pathways include oxidative stress, polyol pathway flux, hexosamine flux, and accumu-lation of AGEs. Hyperglycemia causes nonenzymatic gly-cation of matrix proteins, which subsequently change to irreversible AGEs which bind to AGE receptors on mesan-gial cells and induce cell injury [20]. Glucose can metabo-lize to sorbitol and accumulate in mesangial cells, which leads to nicotinamide adenine dinucleotide phosphate depletion, decreased nitric oxide (NO), increased oxida-tive stress, and activation of protein kinase C (PKC). Phosphorylation of PKC then activates pathways of trans-forming growth factor-β (TGF-β) and vascular endothelial growth factor (VEGF), as well as reactive oxygen species (ROS) and angiotensin II. This causes mesangial expansion

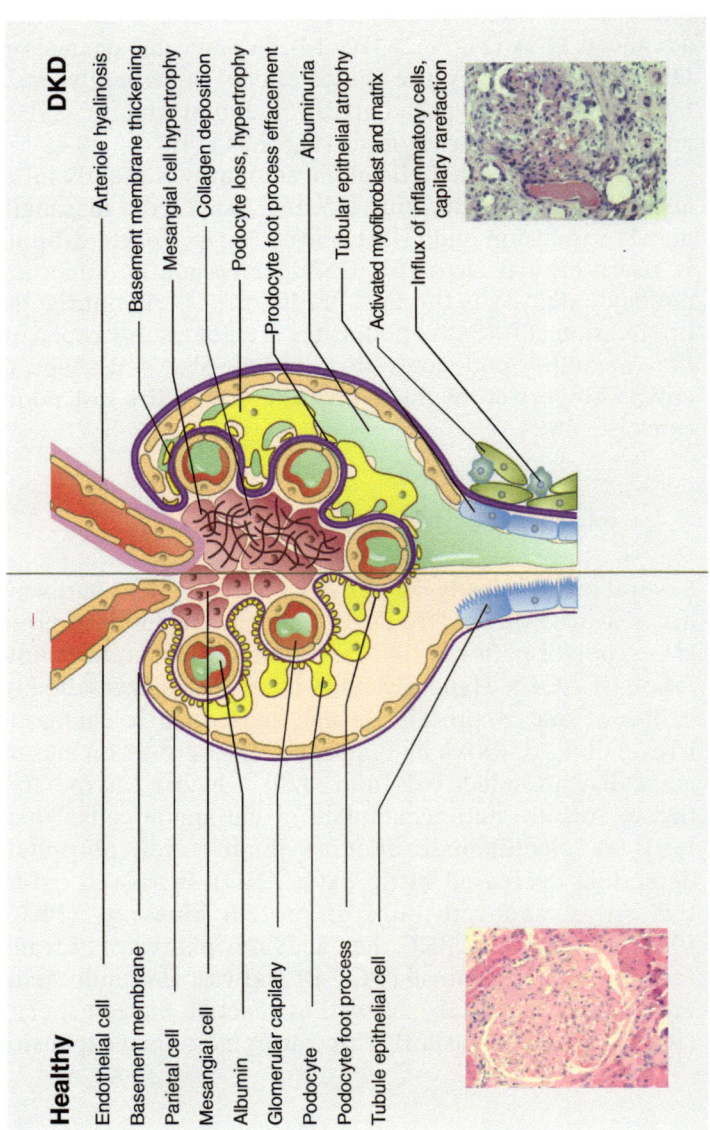

[21, 22]. Increased bioavailability of ROS (oxidative stress) leads to inflammation, fibrosis, and endothelial dysfunction [23, 24]. The identified signaling pathways in the development and progression of DN are summarized in Fig. 2.4 [25].

2.5   Endothelial Dysfunction as a Potential Contributor

Endothelial dysfunction is associated with human DN and diabetic retinopathy. The degree of endothelial dysfunction correlates with the severity of DN in both type 1 and 2 diabetes [26, 27] and is also positively correlated with glomerular injury in patients with type 2 diabetes [28]. Advanced diabetic glomerulopathy often exhibits thrombotic microangiopathy, including glomerular capillary microaneurysms and mesangiolysis, which are typical manifestations of endothelial dysfunction in the glomerulus. In diabetic status, hyperglycemia and other factors cause reduction in the NO levels in the endothelium and contribute to the development of endothelial dysfunction. These factors include increased ROS,

FIGURE 2.2 Pathologic lesions of diabetic kidney disease. The normal healthy glomerulus includes afferent arterioles, capillary loops, endothelial cells, basement membrane, podocytes, parietal epithelial cells, and tubule epithelial cells and is impermeable to albumin. In contrast, the diabetic glomerulus displays arterial hyalinosis, mesangial expansion, collagen deposition, basement membrane thickening, podocyte loss and hypertrophy, albuminuria, tubular epithelial atrophy, accumulation of activated myofibroblasts and matrix, influx of inflammatory cells, and capillary rarefaction. Also shown are a normal healthy human glomerular section and a kidney section from a sample with diabetic kidney disease (PAS stained). 400× original magnification (Reproduced with permission from Reidy et al. [12] © American Society for Clinical Investigation)

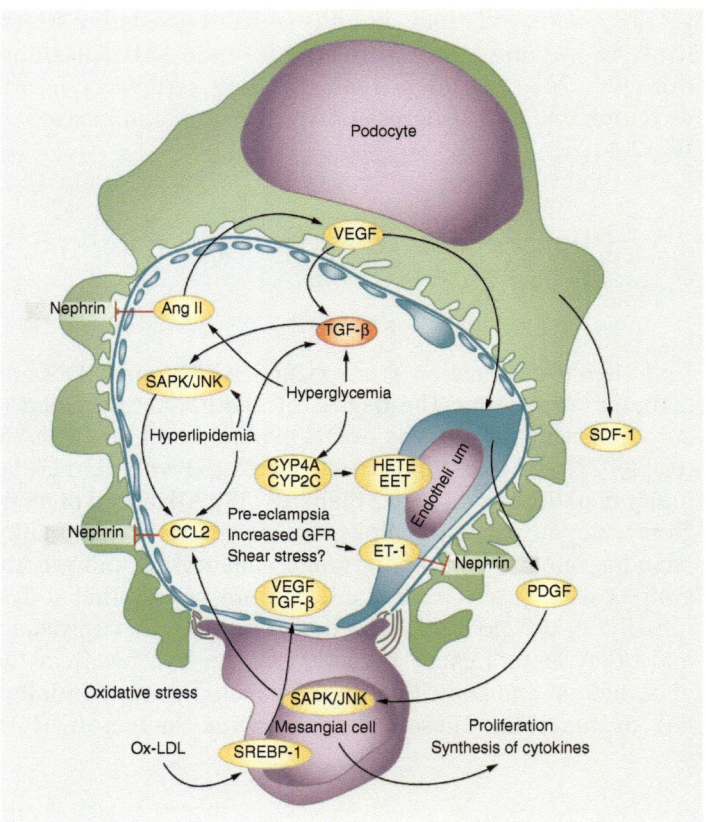

FIGURE 2.3 Mediator for glomerular remodeling. Key mediators of glomerular remodeling in DN. The structural and spatial integrity of the glomerular capillary depends on a podocyte-derived vascular endothelial growth factor (*VEGF*) gradient, synthesis of a basal lamina by podocytes and the endothelium, tensile force exerted on the capillary by contractile mesangial cells, and maintenance of the podocyte slit diaphragm complex of which nephrin is a key component. Hyperglycemia stimulates synthesis of angiotensin II, promotes activation of transforming growth factor (TGF)-β, and induces alterations in CYP4A and CYP2C, which are involved in the synthesis of eicosanoids (e.g., HETE and EET) by endothelial cells. Hyperlipidemia and the associated oxidative stress act through the stress-associated protein kinase subset of MAPK signaling

endothelial nitric oxide synthase (eNOS) inactivation, and an increase of uric acid (Fig. 2.5) [29].

2.6   Inflammatory Pathways

Many factors, such as diet, age, lifestyle, and obesity, are known to contribute to the development of DN. Inflammation has been found to play an essential role in the progression of DN [30, 31]. Evidence from human kidney biopsies has shown that macrophage accumulation in kidneys of patients with diabetes predicts the decline of renal function, suggesting a pathogenic role for these cells in DN [32–34]. These findings are supported in various animal studies in both type 1 and type 2 diabetes [35, 36]. In a type 1 diabetic mouse model (streptozotocin-injected mice), a threefold increase in glomerular and interstitial macrophages was found between 2 and 18 weeks after the onset of diabetes. Macrophage accumulation positively

----

pathways (*SAPK/JNK*) to upregulate expression of cytokines such as CCL2. SAPK/JNK activation also is stimulated by lipid-induced release of TGF-β. Oxidized lipoproteins stimulate the secretion of TGF-β and VEGF by mesangial cells by activation of the SREBP-1 receptor. Alterations in podocyte-derived VEGF gradients, possibly in concert with the systemic VEGF release associated with hyperlipidemia, drive TGF-β activation and endothelial-cell synthesis of PDGF, which in turn further activates mesangial-cell responses. Alterations in glomerular capillary pressure and, perhaps, shear stress, stimulate the synthesis of endothelin-1 by podocytes. Angiotensin II, endothelin-1, and CCL2 have all been shown to downregulate nephrin expression. Activation of TGF-β drives a plethora of glomerular and tubular responses. *Ang II* angiotensin II, *CCL2* chemokine (C–C motif) ligand 2, *CYP4A* cytochrome P450 4A, *CYP2C* cytochrome P450 2C, *EET* epoxyeicosatrienoic acid, *GFR* glomerular filtration rate, *HETE* 20-hydroxyeicosatetraenoic acid, *Ox-LDL* oxidized low-density lipoprotein, *SAP/JNK* stress-activated protein kinase/Jun amino-terminal kinases (Reproduced with permission from Rutledge et al. [14] © Nature)

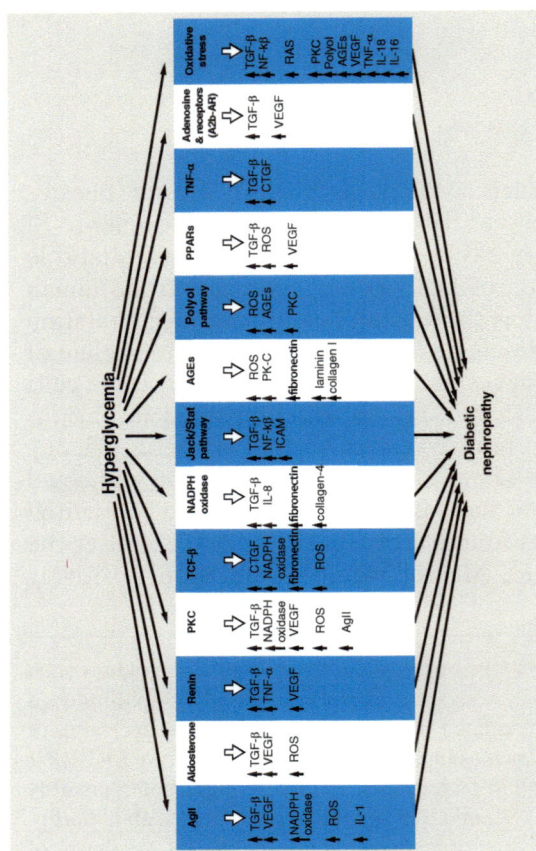

Vasoactive mediators:
R-A system activation
ACE2 modulation
Increased nitrous oxide production
Increased COX-2 derived prostanoids

Systemic factors:
Hyperglycaemia
Systemic hypertension
High protein diet
Obesity

FIGURE 2.4 Tangled web of diabetic nephropathy pathogenesis. Note the pathways, mediators and interference, or overlaps between contributors (Reproduced with permission from Tavafi [25] © Majid Tavafi. Published by Nickan Research Institute) *ACE* angiotensin-converting enzyme; *Ag* angiotensin; *AGE* advanced glycation end-product; *COX* cyclooxygenase; *CTGF* connective tissue growth factor; *ICAM* intercellular adhesion molecule 1; *IL* interleukin; *NADPH* nicotamide adenine dinucleotide phosphate; *NF-κβ* nuclear factor kappa beta; *PKC* protein kinase C; *R-A* renin-aldosterone; *ROS* reactive oxygen species; *TGF* transforming growth factor; *TNF* tumor necrosis factor; *VEGF* vascular endothelial growth factor

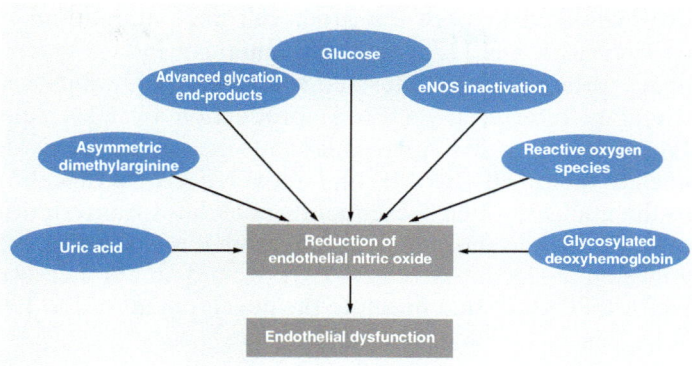

FIGURE 2.5 Factors contributing to endothelial dysfunction. Factors including reactive oxygen species, eNOS inactivation, and uric acid contribute to a reduction in the levels of nitric oxide in the endothelium, which in turn leads to endothelial dysfunction. *eNOS* endothelial nitric oxide synthase (Reproduced with permission from Nakagawa et al. [29] © Nature)

correlated with clinical signs of kidney damage, namely, increased levels of albuminuria and serum creatinine. Histologic analysis of the kidney identified an association between macrophages and pathological changes often present in DN (e.g., glomerular hypertrophy, hypercellularity, tubular atrophy, interstitial myofibroblast accumulation, and collagen IV deposition) [35]. In a type 2 diabetic mouse model (*db/db* mice), 50 % of male mice with diabetes developed a progressive increase in glomerular macrophages (tenfold) and interstitial macrophages (threefold) between 4 and 8 months of age, which correlated with the development of hyperglycemia, albuminuria, and fibrosis, which is also present in DN in humans [36].

Many inflammatory molecules are involved in macrophage infiltration and subsequent kidney injury in diabetic nephropathy. For example, intercellular adhesion molecule-1 (ICAM-1), one of the major molecules involved in leukocyte firm attachment on vascular endothelium, is overexpressed in both the glomeruli and interstitium of patients with DN [37]. Hyperglycemia can induce macrophage production of interleukin (IL)-12 [38], which can stimulate interferon-γ (IFN-γ) production by CD4 cells. Free fatty acids, hyperglycemia, and obesity may activate nuclear factor kB (NF-kB) and allow NF-kB translocation to the nucleus, which subsequently stimulates transcription of genes such as those related to endothelin-1, vascular cell adhesion molecule-1, ICAM-1, IL-6, and tumor necrosis factor-α (TNF-α) that promote the development of DN [39, 40].

Based on the evidence that inflammation plays significant role in the development of DN, many anti-inflammatory drugs have been tried as therapeutics for DN, with different levels of efficacy. For example, pentoxifylline inhibits TNF-α mRNA expression [41]. However, patients treated with pentoxifylline in combination with drugs inhibiting RAAS did not have decreased albuminuria [42, 43]. Inhibition of NF-kB in the kidney using peroxisome proliferator-activated receptor-γ [44] or pentosan polysulfate [45] may ameliorate DN in animal models. However, clear demonstration of the efficacy of inhibition of NF-kB in delaying progression of DN in humans has not been reported. These findings suggest that in humans, different bioactive molecules (not yet identified) may be involved in macrophages and inflammation causing diabetic kidney damage.

2.7   Role of the Renin–Angiotensin– Aldosterone System

Angiotensin II and other components of the RAAS have a central role in DN pathogenesis and progression. As it is an inflammatory condition, angiotensin II levels have been found to be elevated in macrophages and lymphocytes

[46]. Angiotensin II can activate and upregulate NF-kB, causing production of chemokines and leading to further renal damage [47]. Angiotensin II is also localized in tubular-, interstitial-, and fibroblast-like cells, which work together with high glucose and inflammatory mediators to target tubular cells and cause impaired kidney function in diabetes [48]. Increased angiotensin II activity can also cause hypertrophy of mesangial cells and tubular epithelial cells [49] and promote TGF-β production, which can cause glomerular sclerosis. Inhibition of angiotensin II production or activity by angiotensin-converting enzyme (ACE) inhibitors or angiotensin II receptor blockers (ARBs) has renoprotective effects in patients with diabetes.

2.8   Genetic and Epigenetic Factors

Only a subset of individuals living with diabetes (~40 %) develop DN, and studies have shown that this is not just due to poor blood glucose control [50–54]. DN appears to cluster in families, which suggests a shared genetic or environmental contribution to this disease [50]. There is abundant evidence supporting genetic susceptibility to nephropathy in both type 1 and type 2 diabetes. Several consortia have investigated genetic risk factors for DN including:

- Genetics of Kidneys in Diabetes (GoKinD)
- Warren 3 collection
- European rational approach for the genetics of diabetic complications (Euragedic)
- Finnish Diabetic Nephropathy (FinnDiane)
- Family Investigation of Nephropathy and Diabetes (FIND)
- GEnetics of Nephropathy: an Internal Effort (GENIE)
- Surrogate markers for Micro- and Macrovascular hard end points for Innovative diabetes Tools (SUMMIT) [51–54]

Genetic risk factors for DN appear to differ between patients with type 1 and type 2 diabetes, although some overlap has been reported. The GENIE study identified one intronic single nucleotide polymorphism (SNP) in the *ERBB4* gene ($P = 2.1 \times 10^{-7}$) suggestively associated with T1DN and two ESRD-associated SNPs (rs7583877 in the *AFF3* gene; rs12437854 between *RGMA* and *MCTP2* genes) [51]. Functional evidence supports AFF3 as a novel risk factor for ESRD in type 1 diabetes [51], perhaps influencing renal tubule fibrosis via the TGF-β pathway. *FRMD3*, *MYH9-APOL1,* and *ACACB* genes have been identified across multiple studies with supporting functional evidence that SNPs in these genes are important risk factors for type 2 diabetes-related DN [55, 56]. A meta-analysis of DN-associated genetic variants in inflammation and angiogenesis involved in different biochemical pathways was performed, and the results indicate that 11 genetic variants within or near *VEGFA*, *CCR5*, *CCL2*, *IL-1*, *MMP9*, *EPO*, *IL-8*, *ADIPOQ,* and *IL-10* showed significant positive association with DN. Gene ontology or pathway analysis showed that these genes may contribute to the pathophysiology of DN [57].

Most of the genome-wide association studies (GWAS) used GFR or ESRD as outcomes instead of using rates of GFR decline or albuminuria. Thus, loci associated with diabetic albuminuria have not yet been identified [58]. One future option is to use extreme phenotypes for 'enriched' case-control studies where cases of early-onset DN (albuminuria) or rapidly declining renal function (rapidly decreasing GFR) are compared to controls with a long duration of diabetes and no evidence of kidney disease. Over 85 % of the GWAS-identified SNPs are in noncoding regions of the genome. The role of these SNPs in the development and progression of DN still needs to be determined [59]. Through advances in next-generation sequencing technologies and analysis options, more comprehensive analyses of the human genome have become possible. Next-generation genome sequencing provides rich, complementary information on common SNPs, rare SNPs, and copy-number variation [60, 61].

Emerging evidence shows that epigenetic mechanisms in chromatin including histone posttranslational modifications, DNA methylation, and microRNA might also play key roles in the pathogenesis of DN. Transient hyperglycemia can cause Set7/9-mediated histone methylation, which subsequently causes a sustained increase in NF-kB-p65 gene expression in bovine aortic endothelial cells [62] and in a human microvascular endothelial-cell line [63]. Periods of transient or prior hyperglycemia lead to various methylation and demethylation events that, when integrated, have an impact on gene activity. Active NF-kB-p65 gene expression is linked to persisting epigenetic marks that are maintained when the cell is removed from its hyperglycemic environment. The same phenomenon is seen in several randomized clinic trials which demonstrated that the stressors of diabetic vasculature persist even after glycemic control has been achieved [64]. The persistent adverse effects of hyperglycemia on the development and progression of complications have been defined as "metabolic memory." Oxidative stress, AGEs, and epigenetic changes have been implicated in the process.

It is worth mentioning that patients with diabetes mellitus can also be subject to nondiabetic renal disease and may be seen in significant number of patients. Usually there is a giveaway in the form of lack of concurrent retinopathy, rapid decline in renal function in patients with previously stable renal status, heavy proteinuria or renal impairment in patients with diabetes mellitus of less than 5 years duration, and unexplained microscopic hematuria. In these cases, a prompt consultation with a nephrologist is recommended.

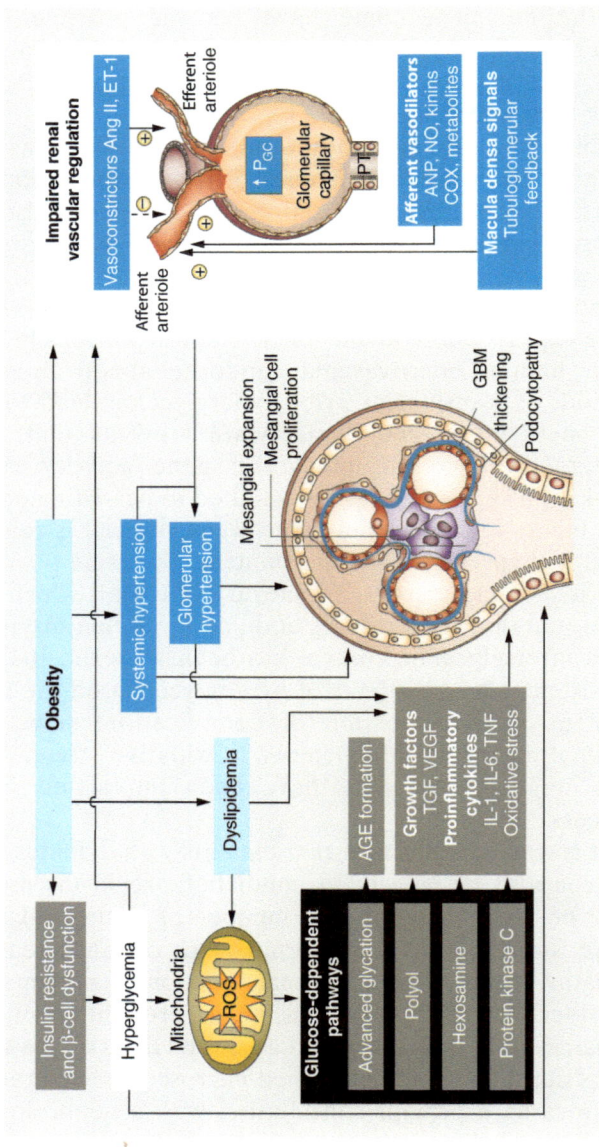

In summary, the pathogenesis of DN is multifactorial, including both genetic and environmental factors (Fig. 2.6) [65]. Hyperglycemia affects patients carrying candidate genes associated with susceptibility to DN and results in metabolic and hemodynamic alterations. Hyperglycemia alters vasoactive regulators of glomerular arteriolar tone and causes glomerular hyperfiltration. Production of AGEs and oxidative stress interacts with various cytokines such as TGF-β and angiotensin II to cause kidney damage. Additionally, oxidative stress can cause endothelial dysfunction and systemic hypertension. Inflammatory pathways are also activated and interact with the other pathways to cause kidney damage.

FIGURE 2.6 Pathogenesis of kidney disease in patients with diabetes. Hemodynamic and metabolic factors, with a central role for chronic hyperglycemia, have pivotal roles in the pathophysiology of diabetic nephropathy. Obesity and chronic hyperglycemia alter vasoactive regulators of afferent and efferent arteriolar tone, leading to increased PGC, hyperperfusion, and hyperfiltration. These early renal hemodynamic changes, combined with systemic hypertension, are important in the development and progression of renal disease in type 2 diabetes mellitus. Additionally, chronic hyperglycemia and dyslipidemia induce mitochondrial superoxide overproduction, which activates several well-defined pathways leading to the development and progression of diabetic nephropathy. Collectively, these factors in the diabetic milieu lead to glomerular damage, histologically characterized by thickening of the glomerular and tubular basement membranes, mesangial expansion, and podocytopathy. *AGE* advanced glycation end products, *Ang II* angiotensin II, *ANP* atrial natriuretic peptide, *COX* cyclooxygenase, *ET-1* endothelin-1, *GBM* glomerular basement membrane, *IL* interleukin, *NO* nitric oxide, *PGC* glomerular capillary hydraulic pressure, *PT* proximal tubule, *ROS* reactive oxygen species, *T2DM* type 2 diabetes mellitus, *TGF* transforming growth factor, *TNF* tumor necrosis factor, *VEGF* vascular endothelial growth factor A (Reproduced with permission from Muskiet et al. [65] © Nature)

References

1. Reutens AT. Epidemiology of diabetic kidney disease. Med Clin North Am. 2013;97:1–18.
2. Eboh C, Chowdhury TA. Management of diabetic renal disease. Ann Transl Med. 2015;3:154.
3. The United States Renal Data System (USRDS). Excerpts from the USRDS 2009 annual data report: atlas of end-stage renal disease in the United States. Am J Kidney Dis. 2010;55:S1.
4. Rudberg S, Osterby R. Decreasing glomerular filtration rate – an indicator of more advanced diabetic glomerulopathy in the early course of microalbuminuria in IDDM adolescents? Nephrol Dial Transplant. 1997;12:1149–54.
5. Nelson RG, Knowler WC, McCance DR, Sievers ML, Pettitt DJ, Charles MA, et al. Determinants of end-stage renal disease in Pima Indians with type 2 (non-insulin-dependent) diabetes mellitus and proteinuria. Diabetologia. 1993;36:1087–93.
6. Amin R, Turner C, van Aken S, Bahu TK, Watts A, Lindsell DRM, et al. The relationship between microalbuminuria and glomerular filtration rate in young type 1 diabetic subjects: The Oxford Regional Prospective Study. Kidney Int. 2005;68:1740–9.
7. Premaratne E, Verma S, Ekinci EI, Theverkalam G, Jerums G, MacIsaac RJ. The impact of hyperfiltration on the diabetic kidney. Diabetes Metab. 2015;41:5–17.
8. Magee GM, Bilous RW, Cardwell CR, Hunter SJ, Kee F, Fogarty DG. Is hyperfiltration associated with the future risk of developing diabetic nephropathy? A meta-analysis. Diabetologia. 2009;52:691–7.
9. Bjornstad P, Cherney DZ, Snell-Bergeon JK, Pyle L, Rewers M, Johnson RJ, et al. Rapid GFR decline is associated with renal hyperfiltration and impaired GFR in adults with Type 1 diabetes. Nephrol Dial Transplant. 2015.
10. Moriya T, Tsuchiya A, Okizaki S, Hayashi A, Tanaka K, Shichiri M. Glomerular hyperfiltration and increased glomerular filtration surface are associated with renal function decline in normo- and microalbuminuric type 2 diabetes. Kidney Int. 2012;81:486–93.
11. Premaratne E, MacIsaac RJ, Tsalamandris C, Panagiotopoulos S, Smith T, Jerums G. Renal hyperfiltration in type 2 diabetes: effect of age-related decline in glomerular filtration rate. Diabetologia. 2005;48:2486–93.

12. Reidy K, Kang HM, Hostetter T, Susztak K. Molecular mechanisms of diabetic kidney disease. J Clin Invest. 2014;124:2333–40.
13. Tervaert TWC, Mooyaart AL, Amann K, Cohen AH, Cook HT, Drachenberg CB, et al. Pathologic classification of diabetic nephropathy. J Am Soc Nephrol. 2010;21:556–63.
14. Rutledge JC, Ng KF, Aung HH, Wilson DW. Role of triglyceride-rich lipoproteins in diabetic nephropathy. Nat Rev Nephrol. 2010;6:361–70.
15. Urizar RE, Schwartz A, Top Jr F, Vernier RL. The nephrotic syndrome in children with diabetes mellitus of recent onset. N Engl J Med. 1969;281:173–81.
16. Fioretto P, Caramori ML, Mauer M. The kidney in diabetes: dynamic pathways of injury and repair. The Camillo Golgi Lecture 2007. Diabetologia. 2008;51:1347–55.
17. Pagtalunan ME, Miller PL, Jumping-Eagle S, Nelson RG, Myers BD, Rennke HG, et al. Podocyte loss and progressive glomerular injury in type II diabetes. J Clin Invest. 1997;99:342–8.
18. Steffes MW, Schmidt D, McCrery R, Basgen JM, International Diabetic Nephropathy Study Group. Glomerular cell number in normal subjects and in type 1 diabetic patients. Kidney Int. 2001;59:2104–13.
19. Romagnani P, Remuzzi G. Renal progenitors in non-diabetic and diabetic nephropathies. Trends Endocrinol Metab. 2013;24:13–20.
20. Singh AK, Mo W, Dunea G, Arruda JA. Effect of glycated proteins on the matrix of glomerular epithelial cells. J Am Soc Nephrol. 1998;9:802–10.
21. Arora MK, Singh UK. Molecular mechanisms in the pathogenesis of diabetic nephropathy: an update. Vascul Pharmacol. 2013;58:259–71.
22. Sung SH, Ziyadeh FN, Wang A, Pyagay PE, Kanwar YS, Chen S. Blockade of vascular endothelial growth factor signaling ameliorates diabetic albuminuria in mice. J Am Soc Nephrol. 2006;17:3093–104.
23. Kaneto H, Katakami N, Kawamori D, Miyatsuka T, Sakamoto K, Matsuoka TA, et al. Involvement of oxidative stress in the pathogenesis of diabetes. Antioxid Redox Signal. 2007;9:355–66.
24. Thallas-Bonke V, Thorpe SR, Coughlan MT, Fukami K, Yap FY, Sourris K, et al. Inhibition of NADPH oxidase prevents advanced glycation end product-mediated damage in diabetic

nephropathy through a protein kinase C-alpha-dependent pathway. Diabetes. 2008;57:460–9.
25. Tavafi M. Complexity of diabetic nephropathy pathogenesis and design of investigations. J Renal Inj Prev. 2013;2:59–62.
26. Stehouwer CD, Stroes ES, Hackeng WH, Mulder PG, Den Ottolander GJ. von Willebrand factor and development of diabetic nephropathy in IDDM. Diabetes. 1991;40:971–6.
27. Stehouwer CD, Nauta JJ, Zeldenrust GC, Hackeng WH, Donker AJ, den Ottolander GJ. Urinary albumin excretion, cardiovascular disease, and endothelial dysfunction in non-insulin-dependent diabetes mellitus. Lancet. 1992;340:319–23.
28. Fioretto P, Stehouwer CD, Mauer M, Chiesura-Corona M, Brocco E, Carraro A, et al. Heterogeneous nature of microalbuminuria in NIDDM: studies of endothelial function and renal structure. Diabetologia. 1998;41:233–6.
29. Nakagawa T, Tanabe K, Croker BP, Johnson RJ, Grant MB, Kosugi T, et al. Endothelial dysfunction as a potential contributor in diabetic nephropathy. Nat Rev Nephrol. 2011;7:36–44.
30. Rivero A, Mora C, Muros M, Garcia J, Herrera H, Navarro-Gonzalez JF. Pathogenic perspectives for the role of inflammation in diabetic nephropathy. Clin Sci (Lond). 2009;116:479–92.
31. Navarro-Gonzalez JF, Mora-Fernandez C, Muros de Fuentes M, Garcia-Perez J. Inflammatory molecules and pathways in the pathogenesis of diabetic nephropathy. Nature Rev Nephrol. 2011;7:327–40.
32. Furuta T, Saito T, Ootaka T, Soma J, Obara K, Abe K, et al. The role of macrophages in diabetic glomerulosclerosis. Am J Kidney Dis. 1993;21:480–5.
33. Nguyen D, Ping F, Mu W, Hill P, Atkins RC, Chadban SJ. Macrophage accumulation in human progressive diabetic nephropathy. Nephrology (Carlton). 2006;11:226–31.
34. Yonemoto S, Machiguchi T, Nomura K, Minakata T, Nanno M, Yoshida H. Correlations of tissue macrophages and cytoskeletal protein expression with renal fibrosis in patients with diabetes mellitus. Clin Exp Nephrol. 2006;10:186–92.
35. Chow FY, Nikolic-Paterson DJ, Atkins RC, Tesch GH. Macrophages in streptozotocin-induced diabetic nephropathy: potential role in renal fibrosis. Nephrol Dial. 2004;19:2987–96.
36. Chow F, Ozols E, Nikolic-Paterson DJ, Atkins RC, Tesch GH. Macrophages in mouse type 2 diabetic nephropathy: correlation with diabetic state and progressive renal injury. Kidney Int. 2004;65:116–28.

37. Hirata K, Shikata K, Matsuda M, Akiyama K, Sugimoto H, Kushiro M, et al. Increased expression of selectins in kidneys of patients with diabetic nephropathy. Diabetologia. 1998;41:185–92.
38. Wen YS, Gu JL, Li SL, Reddy MA, Natarajan R, Nadler JL. Elevated glucose and diabetes promote interleukin-12 cytokine gene expression in mouse macrophages. Endocrinology. 2006;147:2518–25.
39. Ha HJ, Yu MR, Choi YJ, Kitamura M, Lee HB. Role of high glucose-induced nuclear factor-kappa B activation in monocyte chemoattractant protein-1 expression by mesangial cells. J Am Soc Nephrol. 2002;13:894–902.
40. Chen JS, Lee HS, Jin JS, Chen A, Lin SH, Ka SM, et al. Attenuation of mouse mesangial cell contractility by high glucose and mannitol: Involvement of protein kinase C and focal adhesion kinase. J Biomed Sci. 2004;11:142–51.
41. Han J, Thompson P, Beutler B. Dexamethasone and pentoxifylline inhibit endotoxin-induced cachectin/tumor necrosis factor synthesis at separate points in the signaling pathway. J Exp Med. 1990;172:391–4.
42. Badri S, Dashti-Khavidaki S, Lessan-Pezeshki M, Abdollahi M. A review of the potential benefits of pentoxifylline in diabetic and non-diabetic proteinuria. J Pharm Pharm Sci. 2011;14:128–37.
43. Perkins RM, Aboudara MC, Uy AL, Olson SW, Cushner HM, Yuan CM. Effect of pentoxifylline on GFR decline in CKD: a pilot, double-blind, randomized, placebo-controlled trial. Am J Kidney Dis. 2009;53:606–16.
44. Makino H, Miyamoto Y, Sawai K, Mori K, Mukoyama M, Nakao K, et al. Altered gene expression related to glomerulogenesis and podocyte structure in early diabetic nephropathy of db/db mice and its restoration by pioglitazone. Diabetes. 2006;55:2747–56.
45. Wu J, Guan TJ, Zheng SR, Grosjean F, Liu WC, Xiong HB, et al. Inhibition of inflammation by pentosan polysulfate impedes the development and progression of severe diabetic nephropathy in aging C57B6 mice. Lab Invest. 2011;91:1459–71.
46. Rodriguez-Iturbe B, Pons H, Herrera-Acosta J, Johnson RJ. Role of immunocompetent cells in nonimmune renal diseases. Kidney Int. 2001;59:1626–40.
47. Ruiz-Ortega M, Lorenzo O, Ruperez M, Esteban V, Mezzano S, Egido J. Renin-angiotensin system and renal damage: emerging

data on angiotensin II as a proinflammatory mediator. Contrib Nephrol. 2001;135:123–37.

48. Mezzano S, Droguett A, Burgos ME, Ardiles LG, Flores CA, Aros CA, et al. Renin-angiotensin system activation and interstitial inflammation in human diabetic nephropathy. Kidney Int Suppl. 2003;86:S64–70.

49. Wolf G, Mueller E, Stahl RA, Ziyadeh FN. Angiotensin II-induced hypertrophy of cultured murine proximal tubular cells is mediated by endogenous transforming growth factor-beta. J Clin Invest. 1993;92:1366–72.

50. Seaquist ER, Goetz FC, Rich S, Barbosa J. Familial clustering of diabetic kidney disease. Evidence for genetic susceptibility to diabetic nephropathy. N Engl J Med. 1989;320:1161–5.

51. Sandholm N, Salem RM, McKnight AJ, Brennan EP, Forsblom C, Isakova T, et al. New susceptibility loci associated with kidney disease in type 1 diabetes. PLoS Genet. 2012;8, e1002921.

52. Mueller PW, Rogus JJ, Cleary PA, Zhao Y, Smiles AM, Steffes MW, et al. Genetics of Kidneys in Diabetes (GoKinD) study: a genetics collection available for identifying genetic susceptibility factors for diabetic nephropathy in type 1 diabetes. J Am Soc Nephrol. 2006;17:1782–90.

53. Igo Jr RP, Iyengar SK, Nicholas SB, Goddard KA, Langefeld CD, Hanson RL, et al., Family Investigation of Nephropathy and Diabetes Research Group. Genomewide linkage scan for diabetic renal failure and albuminuria: the FIND study. Am J Nephrol. 2011;33:381–9.

54. Tarnow L, Groop PH, Hadjadj S, Kazeem G, Cambien F, Marre M, et al. European rational approach for the genetics of diabetic complications – EURAGEDIC: patient populations and strategy. Nephrol Dial Transplant. 2008;23:161–8.

55. Freedman BI, Langefeld CD, Lu L, Divers J, Comeau ME, Kopp JB, et al. Differential effects of MYH9 and APOL1 risk variants on FRMD3 association with diabetic ESRD in African Americans. PLoS Genet. 2011;7:e1002150.

56. Maeda S, Kobayashi MA, Araki S, Babazono T, Freedman BI, Bostrom MA, et al. A single nucleotide polymorphism within the acetyl-coenzyme A carboxylase beta gene is associated with proteinuria in patients with type 2 diabetes. PLoS Genet. 2010;6:e1000842.

57. Nazir N, Siddiqui K, Al-Qasim S, Al-Naqeb D. Meta-analysis of diabetic nephropathy associated genetic variants in inflammation

and angiogenesis involved in different biochemical pathways. BMC Med Genet. 2014;15:103.

58. Kottgen A, Pattaro C, Boger CA, Fuchsberger C, Olden M, Glazer NL, et al. New loci associated with kidney function and chronic kidney disease. Nat Genet. 2010;42:376–84.

59. Maurano MT, Humbert R, Rynes E, Thurman RE, Haugen E, Wang H, et al. Systematic localization of common disease-associated variation in regulatory DNA. Science. 2012; 337:1190–5.

60. Ng SB, Buckingham KJ, Lee C, Bigham AW, Tabor HK, Dent KM, et al. Exome sequencing identifies the cause of a mendelian disorder. Nat Genet. 2010;42:30–5.

61. Ng SB, Turner EH, Robertson PD, Flygare SD, Bigham AW, Lee C, et al. Targeted capture and massively parallel sequencing of 12 human exomes. Nature. 2009;461:272–6.

62. El-Osta A, Brasacchio D, Yao D, Pocai A, Jones PL, Roeder RG, Cooper ME, Brownlee M. Transient high glucose causes persistent epigenetic changes and altered gene expression during subsequent normoglycemia. J Exp Med. 2008;205:2409–17.

63. Brasacchio D, Okabe J, Tikellis C, Balcerczyk A, George P, Baker EK, et al. Hyperglycemia induces a dynamic cooperativity of histone methylase and demethylase enzymes associated with gene-activating epigenetic marks that coexist on the lysine tail. Diabetes. 2009;58:12–1236.

64. Zhang E, Wu Y. Metabolic memory: mechanisms and implications for diabetic vasculopathies. Sci China Life Sci. 2014;57:845–51.

65. Muskiet MH, Smits MM, Morsink LM, Diamant M. The gut-renal axis: do incretin-based agents confer renoprotection in diabetes? Nat Rev Nephrol. 2014;10:88–103.

Chapter 3
Patient Assessment and Diagnosis

Daisuke Koya

3.1   Introduction

The 2015 International Diabetes Federation Atlas reported that 415 million people live with diabetes worldwide, and 642 million people will have diabetes worldwide by 2040 [1]. Long-term disease results in vascular changes and dysfunction, which are major causes of morbidity and mortality in patients with diabetes. Among diabetic vascular complications, diabetic nephropathy (DN) is a leading cause of chronic kidney disease (CKD) and end-stage renal disease (ESRD) [2]. Moderately and severely increased albuminuria and a decline in the glomerular filtration rate (GFR) are early markers of CKD and are recognized as independent risk factors for the development of ESRD and the onset of cardiovascular diseases (CVD). Therefore, the early assessment of DN in patients with diabetes is critical.

The pathogenesis of DN is complex and has not yet been completely elucidated (see Chap. 2). Hyperglycemia is a major factor, and high systemic blood and intraglomerular pressure (in association with renin-angiotensin system [RAS] activation), certain inflammatory cytokines and growth factors, and dyslipidemia all contribute to DN pathogenesis [3–5]. Current therapeutic strategies, such as controlling blood glucose (HbA1c) and blood pressure, have demonstrated efficacy in landmark clinical trials [6]. It has been shown that a reduction in moderate and severely increased albuminuria (referred to as remission or regression) was more likely to occur than progression to overt proteinuria when clinicians employed a multifactorial control approach to reduce both renal and cardiovascular risk factors [7].

This chapter will focus on the current standard assessment and diagnosis of DN (especially in the early stages) and strategies to prevent progression. In addition, markers used predict the early decline of renal function in patients with diabetes but without severely increased albuminuria, such as urinary liver-type fatty acid-binding protein (L-FABP), urinary type IV collagen, and circulating tumor necrosis factor receptors (TNFR) 1 and 2 will also be discussed.

3.2   Assessment of Albuminuria and Renal Function

An early clinical sign of DN is moderately increased urinary albumin excretion, referred to as microalbuminuria and defined as a urine albumin/creatinine (Cr) ratio (ACR) $\geq$30 mg/g Cr in a random untimed urine sample with a subsequent early morning urine sample [8]. Moderately increased urinary albumin excretion that progresses to severely increased albuminuria is referred to as macroalbuminuria or overt proteinuria and, in some cases, results in nephrotic range albuminuria (ACR >2200 mg/g). Severely increased albuminuria is defined as an ACR $\geq$ 300 mg/g Cr; it leads to a decline in renal function, which is defined in terms of the GFR [8] and generally progresses to ESRD 6–8 years after the onset of overt proteinuria [9]. The ACR should be confirmed in the absence of urinary tract infection, intensive physical activity, fever, congestive heart failure, hyperglycemia, and higher systolic blood pressure in two additional first-void specimens collected during the following 3–6 months [8].

To assess renal function, the Kidney Disease: Improving Global Outcomes (KDIGO) CKD working group recommends using serum creatinine (SCr) and a GFR estimating equation for the initial assessment, which is referred to as the estimated GFRcreat (or eGFRcreat) [8]. In circumstances where estimated glomerular filtration rate (eGFR) is based on serum creatinine and is considered less accurate, the KDIGO CKD working group suggests measuring cystatin C and using a GFR-estimating equation referred to as the eGFRcys [8]. Based on the combined assessment of albuminuria and the eGFR, the categories of DN can be used to predict the risk of its progression, as well as the development of CVD and mortality [8] (Fig. 3.1).

Microalbuminuria in patients with diabetes has been recognized as a useful biomarker for the diagnosis of early-stage DN and as a predictive factor for progression to ESRD, as well as

Composite ranking for relative risks by GFR and albuminuria (KDIGO 2009)			Albuminuria stages, description and range (mg/g)				
			A1		A2	A3	
			Optimal and high-normal		High	Very high and nephrotic	
			<10	10-29	30-299	300-1999	≥2000
GFR stages, description and range (mL/min per 1.73m²)	G1	High and optimal	>105				
			90-104				
	G2	Mild	75-89				
			60-74				
	G3a	Mild-moderate	45-59				
	G3b	Moderate-severe	30-44				
	G4	Severe	15-29				
	G5	Kidney failure	<15				

FIGURE 3.1 KDIGO 2012 clinical practice guideline for the evaluation and management of chronic kidney disease: composite ranking for relative risks by glomerular filtration rate (*GFR*) and albuminuria. The highest level of albuminuria is termed "nephrotic" to correspond with nephrotic range albuminuria (≥2000 mg/g). *KDIGO* Kidney Disease: Improving Global Outcomes (Reproduced with permission from Levey et al. [8] ©Elsevier)

the risk for future cardiovascular events. In most patients with diabetes, CKD should be attributed to diabetes if any of the following are true: macroalbuminuria is present; microalbuminuria is present alongside diabetic retinopathy; and/or type 1 diabetes has been present for a duration of at least 10 years [8]. However, other causes of CKD should be considered in the presence of the following circumstances:

- diabetic retinopathy is absent;
- GFR is low or rapidly decreasing;
- increasing proteinuria;
- evidence of nephrotic syndrome;
- refractory hypertension;
- active urinary sediments;
- signs or symptoms of other systemic diseases;
- a >30 % reduction in the eGFR has occurred within 2–3 months after the initiation of treatment with an angiotensin-converting enzyme (ACE) inhibitor or an angiotensin II receptor blocker (ARB) [8].

Additionally, microalbuminuria has been shown to be closely associated with an increased risk of cardiovascular morbidity and mortality [10–12]. In a sub-analysis of the UK Prospective Diabetes Study (UKPDS), cardiovascular mortality of patients with type 2 diabetes with microalbuminuria was shown to be two times higher than that of patients with normoalbuminuria [13]. Therefore, microalbuminuria is not only a biomarker for the early diagnosis of DN but also an important therapeutic target for improving the prognosis of renal and cardiovascular risk in patients with diabetes.

3.3   Urinary Liver-Type Fatty Acid-Binding Protein and Type IV Collagen

L-FABP is an intracellular carrier protein of free fatty acids, and it is expressed in the liver and kidney. L-FABP expression occurs in the proximal tubules of the kidney.

Higher urinary L-FABP levels have been associated with renal tubulointerstitial damage because filtered free fatty acids from glomeruli are reabsorbed into the proximal tubules and induce tubulointerstitial damage [14–16]. An observational study in patients with type 2 diabetes with micro- and normoalbuminuria revealed that higher urinary levels of L-FABP were associated with renal function decline and a higher incidence rate of CVD [17]. These findings suggest that urinary L-FABP can be used as a biomarker for predicting future renal function decline and the development of CVD in patients with type 2 diabetes with early-stage nephropathy in addition to albuminuria (Table 3.1) [18, 19].

DN is characterized structurally by the accumulation of mesangial matrix and thickening of the basement membrane in the glomeruli [20], as well as by renal tubular hypertrophy and the associated basement membrane thickening in the tubulointerstitium, followed by tubulointerstitial fibrosis [21]. Excess production of extracellular matrix proteins, such as type IV collagen, could be responsible for these pathologies [22]. Urinary type IV collagen excretion in patients with diabetes has been shown to increase in parallel with urinary albumin levels [23–28]. Thus, a high level of urinary type IV collagen has been proposed as a marker of development and progression of early DN.

Although the median levels of urinary type IV collagen are higher in patients with comorbid diabetes and microalbuminuria than in those with normoalbuminuria, studies have revealed that in patients with normoalbuminuria, urinary type IV collagen levels are still high [29]. Therefore, urinary type IV collagen could be increased before an increase in albuminuria occurs and act as a useful marker for the identification of the early stages of DN. A recent finding failed to show any predictive role of urinary type IV collagen in the development or progression of DN, although the urinary ACR is a highly variable quantity [29]. This result suggests that the increase in urinary type IV collagen in the patients without overt proteinuria could reflect other renal damage

TABLE 3.1 Assessment of albuminuria and renal function: glomerular filtration rate (GFR)

Yearly measurement of urine albumin/g creatinine ratio in patients with type 1 diabetes with duration of >5 years and in all patients with type 2 diabetes:	<30 mg/g: Normal albuminuria ≥30 mg/g: Increased albuminuria >300 mg/g: Severely increased albuminuria >2200 mg/g: Nephrotic rage of albuminuria

Determine estimated glomerular filtration rate (eGFR):

Serum creatinine based	Serum cystatin C based
2009 CKD-EPI creatinine equation: $GFR = 141 * min(Scr/\kappa, 1)\alpha * max(Scr/\kappa, 1)^{-1.209} * 0.993Age * 1.018$ [*if female*] $* 1.159$ [*if black*] Scr is serum creatinine (mg/dL), κ is 0.7 for females and 0.9 for males, α is −0.329 for females and −0.411 for males, min indicates the minimum of Scr/κ or 1, and max indicates the maximum of Scr/κ or 1, age in years	*2012 CKD-EPI cystatin C equation*: $eGFR = 133 * min(Scys/0.8, 1)^{-0.499} * max(ScysC/0.8, 1)^{-1.328} * 0.996Age$ [*0.932 if female*] Scys is standardized serum cystatin C = mg/L, min indicates the minimum of Scys/0.8 or 1, max indicates the maximum of Scys/0.8 or 1, age in years.

Adapted from Levey et al. [18] and Inker et al. [19]

processes not directly related to the degree of albuminuria [29]. The level of urinary type IV collagen is higher in patients with microalbuminuria than in those with normoalbuminuria and was correlated with the level of urinary β_2-microglobulin, diastolic blood pressure, eGFR, and ACR at baseline. In addition, the level of urinary type IV collagen at baseline was inversely correlated with the annual decline in the eGFR during the follow-up period, whereas these levels were not associated with worsening of the stage of DN [29]. Furthermore, the annual decline in the eGFR of patients with increased urinary type IV collagen excretion was greater regardless of the stage of DN [29].

3.3.1   Serum Tumor Necrosis Factor Receptors 1 and 2

Chronic subclinical inflammation is responsible for the development of microalbuminuria in patients with diabetes [30]. Indeed, cross-sectional studies have reported higher levels of inflammation markers, such as high-sensitivity C-reactive protein (hs-CRP), TNF-α, and interleukin-1, in patients with diabetes and DN than in those without DN [31–33]. Interestingly, the Joslin group has reported that the risk of ESRD is associated with higher concentrations of circulating TNFR1 and TNFR2, but not with the other TNF pathway markers (e.g., free or total TNF-α) in patients with type 2 diabetes without proteinuria [34]. Furthermore, Krolewski and colleagues recently reported that elevated TNFR concentrations are inversely associated with renal pathology markers, such as the percentage of endothelial cell fenestration and the total filtration surface per glomerulus, and positively associated with the mesangial fractional volume, glomerular basement membrane width, podocyte foot process width, and percentage of global glomerular sclerosis [35]. Even in homogenous type 1 diabetes without proteinuria and with normal renal function, the same group revealed that higher serum concentrations of TNFR1 and TNFR2 are strongly associated with early renal function decline and progression to CKD3 or a higher stage [36]. Thus, TNFR1 and 2 serum levels could be a prognostic marker used to detect early GFR decline in patients with diabetes who do not first develop albuminuria (Table 3.2) [37].

TABLE 3.2 Supplementary assessment of early glomerular filtration rate (GFR) decline

Additional diagnostic criteria for early GFR decline	
Urinary L-FABP	>8.5 μg/g creatinine
Urinary type IV collagen	>7.3 μg/g creatinine
Circulating TNFR1 and TNFR2 levels	Elevated (varies according to population)

L-FABP, liver-type fatty binding protein; *TNFR*, tumor necrosis factor receptor

References

1. International Diabetes Federation (IDF). IDF diabetes atlas update 2015. www.diabetesatlas.org/resources/2015-atlas.html. Accessed February 2, 2016.
2. Packham DK, Alves TP, Dwyer JP, Atkins R, de Zeeuw D, Cooper M, et al. Relative incidence of ESRD versus cardiovascular mortality in proteinuric type 2 diabetes and nephropathy: results from the DIAMETRIC (Diabetes Mellitus Treatment for Renal Insufficiency Consortium) database. Am J Kidney Dis. 2012;59:75–83.
3. Kitada M, Zhang Z, Mima A, King GL. Molecular mechanisms of diabetic vascular complications. J Diabetes Investig. 2010;1:77–89.
4. Forbes JM, Cooper ME. Mechanisms of diabetic complications. Physiol Rev. 2013;93:137–88.
5. Giunti S, Barit D, Cooper ME. Mechanisms of diabetic nephropathy: role of hypertension. Hypertension. 2006;48:519–26.
6. Koya D, Araki S-I, Haneda M. Therapeutic management of diabetic kidney disease. J Diabetes Investig. 2011;4:248–54.
7. Araki S, Haneda M, Koya D, Kashiwagi A, Uzu T, Kikkawa R. Clinical impact of reducing microalbuminuria in patients with type 2 diabetes mellitus. Diabetes Res Clin Pract. 2008;Suppl 1:S54–8.
8. Levey AS, de Jong PE, Coresh J, Nahas MEI, Astor BC, Matsushita K, et al. The definition, classification, and prognosis of chronic kidney disease: a KDIGO controversies conference report. Kidney Int. 2011;80:17–28.
9. Gross JL, de Azevedo MJ, Silveiro SP, Canani LH, Caramori ML, Zelmanovitz T. Diabetic nephropathy: diagnosis, prevention, and treatment. Diabetes Care. 2005;28:164–76.
10. Garg JP, Bakris GL. Microalbuminuria: marker of vascular dysfunction, risk factor for cardiovascular disease. Vasc Med. 2002;7:35–43.
11. Lane JT. Microalbuminuria as a marker of cardiovascular and renal risk in type 2 diabetes mellitus: a temporal perspective. Am J Physiol Renal Physiol. 2004;286:F442–50.
12. Basi S, Lewis JB. Microalbuminuria as a target to improve cardiovascular and renal outcomes. Am J Kidney Dis. 2006;47:927–46.
13. Adler AI, Stevens RJ, Manley SE, Bilous RW, Cull CA, Holman RR. Development and progression of nephropathy in type 2 diabetes: the United Kingdom Prospective Diabetes Study (UKPDS 64). Kidney Int. 2003;63:225–32.

14. Maatman RG, Van Kuppevelt TH, Veerkamp JH. Two types of fatty acid-binding protein in human kidney. Isolation, characterization and localization. Biochem J. 1991;273:759–76.
15. Thomas ME, Schreiner GF. Contribution of proteinuria to progressive renal injury: consequences of tubular uptake of fatty acid bearing albumin. Am J Nephrol. 1993;13:385–98.
16. Kamijo A, Kimura K, Sugaya T, Yamanouchi M, Hase H, Kaneko T, et al. Urinary free fatty acids bound to albumin aggravate tubulointerstitial damage. Kidney Int. 2002;62:1628–37.
17. Araki S, Haneda M, Koya D, Sugaya T, Isshiki K, Kume S, et al. Predictive effects of urinary liver-type fatty acid-binding protein for deteriorating renal function and incidence of cardiovascular disease in type 2 diabetic patients without advanced nephropathy. Diabetes Care. 2013;36:1248–53.
18. Levey AS, Stevens LA, Schmid CH, Zhang YL, Castro 3rd AF, Feldman HI, et al. A new equation to estimate glomerular filtration rate. Ann Intern Med. 2009;150:604–12.
19. Inker LA, Schmid CH, Tighiouart H, Eckfeldt JH, Feldman HI, Greene T, et al. Estimating glomerular filtration rate from serum creatinine and cystatin C. N Engl J Med. 2012;367:20–9.
20. Najafian B, Mauer M. Progression of diabetic nephropathy in type 1 diabetic patients. Diabetes Res Clin Pract. 2009;83:1–8.
21. Ziyadeh FN. Significance of tubulointerstitial changes in diabetic renal disease. Kidney Int Suppl. 1996;54:S10–3.
22. Suzuki D, Miyazaki M, Jinde K, Koji T, Yagame M, Endoh M, et al. In situ hybridization studies of matrix metalloproteinase-3, tissue inhibitor of metalloproteinase-1 and type IV collagen in diabetic nephropathy. Kidney Int. 1997;52:111–21.
23. Kado S, Aoki A, Wada S, Katayama Y, Kugai N, Yoshizawa N, et al. Urinary type IV collagen as a marker for early diabetic nephropathy. Diabetes Res Clin Pract. 1996;31:103–8.
24. Yagame M, Suzuki D, Jinde K, Saotome N, Sato H, Noguchi M, et al. Significance of urinary type IV collagen in patients with diabetic nephropathy using a highly sensitive one-step sandwich enzyme immunoassay. J Clin Lab Anal. 1997;11:110–6.
25. Kotajima N, Kimura T, Kanda T, Obata K, Kuwabara A, Fukumura Y, et al. Type IV collagen as an early marker for diabetic nephropathy in non-insulin-dependent diabetes mellitus. J Diabetes Complications. 2000;14:13–7.
26. Watanabe H, Sanada H, Shigetomi S, Katoh T, Watanabe T. Urinary excretion of type IV collagen as a specific indicator of the progression of diabetic nephropathy. Nephron. 2000;86:27–35.

27. Cohen MP, Lautenslager GT, Shearman CW. Increased collagen IV excretion in diabetes. A marker of compromised filtration function. Diabetes Care. 2001;24:914–8.
28. Tomino Y, Suzuki S, Azushima C, Shou I, Iijima T, Yagame M, et al. Asian multicenter trials on urinary type IV collagen in patients with diabetic nephropathy. J Clin Lab Anal. 2001;15:188–92.
29. Araki S, Haneda M, Koya D, Isshiki K, Kume S, Sugimoto T, et al. Association between urinary type IV collagen level and deterioration of renal function in type 2 diabetic patients without overt proteinuria. Diabetes Care. 2010;33:1805–10.
30. Navarro-González J, Mora-Fernández C. The role of inflammatory cytokines in diabetic nephropathy. J Am Soc Nephrol. 2008;19:433–42.
31. Flyvbjerg A. Diabetic angiopathy, the complement system and the tumor necrosis factor superfamily. Nat Rev Endocrinol. 2010;6:94–101.
32. Zoppini G, Faccini G, Muggeo M, Zenari L, Falezza G, Targher G. Elevated plasma levels of soluble receptors of TNF-alpha and their association with smoking and microvascular complications in young adults with type 1 diabetes. J Clin Endocrinol Metab. 2001;86:3805–8.
33. Halwachs G, Tiran A, Reisinger EC, Zach R, Sabin K, Fölsch B, et al. Serum levels of the soluble receptor for tumor necrosis factor in patients with renal disease. Clin Investig. 1994;72:473–6.
34. Pavkov ME, Nelson RG, Knowler WC, Cheng Y, Krolewski AS, Niewczas MA. Elevation of circulating TNF receptors 1 and 2 increases the risk of end-stage renal disease in American Indians with type 2 diabetes. Kidney Int. 2015;87:812–9.
35. Pavkov ME, Weil EJ, Fufaa GD, Nelson RG, Lemley KV, Knowler WC, et al. Tumor necrosis factor receptors 1 and 2 are associated with early glomerular lesions in type 2 diabetes. Kidney Int. 2016;89:226–34.
36. Gohda T, Niewczas MA, Ficociello LH, Walker WH, Skupien J, Rosetti F, et al. Circulating TNF receptors 1 and 2 predict stage 3 CKD in type 1 diabetes. J Am Soc Nephrol. 2012;23:516–24.
37. Krolewski AS. Progressive renal decline: the new paradigm of diabetic nephropathy in type 1 diabetes. Diabetes Care. 2015;38:954–62.

Chapter 4
Management of Diabetes in the Pre-End-Stage Renal Disease and Chronic Kidney Disease

Mark Molitch and Allison Hahr

4.1 Introduction

Diabetic kidney disease (DKD) affects approximately 20–40 % of individuals who have diabetes [1]. Given the frequency of nephropathy, it is important to understand the safe use of diabetes medications in this population. Glycemic control in chronic kidney disease (CKD) adds a level of complexity that requires detailed knowledge of which medications can be safely used and how kidney disease affects their metabolism. Additionally, glycemic targets should be individualized for each patient.

4.2 Medications to Treat Diabetes Mellitus in the Presence of Chronic Kidney Disease

There are several different classes of medications available for glycemic control. Please refer to Table 4.1 for dosing adjustments for diabetes medications in the presence of CKD.

G.L. Bakris et al., *Managing Diabetic Nephropathies in Clinical Practice*, DOI 10.1007/978-3-319-08873-0_4, © Springer International Publishing Switzerland 2017

TABLE 4.1 Dose adjustment for insulin and medications for diabetes in pre-end-stage renal disease (ESRD)

Medication class	CKD stages 3 and 4 and pre-dialysis stage 5
Insulin	
Glargine	No advised dose adjustment[a]
Degludec	No advised dose adjustment[a]
Detemir	No advised dose adjustment[a]
NPH	No advised dose adjustment[a]
Regular	No advised dose adjustment[a]
Aspart	No advised dose adjustment[a]
Lispro	No advised dose adjustment[a]
Glulisine	No advised dose adjustment[a]
Inhaled insulin	No advised dose adjustment[a]
Biguanides	
Metformin	Per FDA, Metformin can be used down to eGFR 30 *Consider*: eGFR[b] $\geq$45–59: use caution with dose and follow renal function closely (every 3–6 months) eGFR $\geq$30–44: max dose 1000 mg/day or use 50 % dose reduction. Follow renal function every 3 months. Do not start as new therapy eGFR <30: avoid use
Second-generation sulfonylureas	
Glipizide	eGFR <30: use with caution
Glimepiride	eGFR <60: use with caution eGFR <30: avoid use
Glyburide	Avoid use

TABLE 4.1 (continued)

Medication class	CKD stages 3 and 4 and pre-dialysis stage 5
Glinides	
Repaglinide	No dose adjustment but may wish to use caution with an eGFR <30
Nateglinide	eGFR <60: avoid use (but may consider use if patient is on hemodialysis)
Thiazolidinediones	
Pioglitazone	No dose adjustment
Rosiglitazone	No dose adjustment
Alpha-glucosidase inhibitors	
Acarbose	serum Cr >2 mg/dL: avoid use
Miglitol	eGFR <25 or serum Cr >2 mg/dL: avoid use
DPP-4 inhibitor	
Sitagliptin	eGFR ≥50: 100 mg daily eGFR 30–49: 50 mg daily eGFR <30: 25 mg daily
Saxagliptin	eGFR >50: 2.5 or 5 mg daily GFR ≤50: 2.5 mg daily
Linagliptin	No dose adjustment
Alogliptin	eGFR >60: 25 mg daily eGFR 30–59: 12.5 mg daily eGFR <30: 6.25 mg daily
SGLT2 inhibitors	
Canagliflozin	eGFR 45 to <60: max dose 100 mg once daily eGFR <45: avoid use
Dapagliflozin	eGFR <60: avoid use
Empagliflozin	eGFR <45: avoid use
Dopamine receptor agonist	
Bromocriptine mesylate	No dose adjustment known but not studied: use with caution

(continued)

TABLE 4.1 (continued)

Medication class	CKD stages 3 and 4 and pre-dialysis stage 5
Bile acid sequestrant	
Colesevelam	No dose adjustment known but limited data
GLP-1 agonists	
Exenatide	eGFR 30–50: use caution eGFR <30: avoid use
Liraglutide	No dose adjustment but use caution when starting or titrating the dose
Albiglutide	No dose adjustment needed
Dulaglutide	No dose adjustment needed
Amylin analog	
Pramlintide	No dose adjustment known but not studied in end-stage renal disease

CKD chronic kidney disease, *Cr* creatinine, *DPP-4* dipeptidyl peptidase-4 inhibitor, *eGFR* estimated glomerular filtration rate, *FDA* Food and Drug Administration (United States), *GLP-1* glucagon-like peptide-1, *NPH* neutral protamine Hagedorn, *SGLT2* sodium–glucose cotransporter 2
[a]Adjust dose based on patient response
[b]Units for eGFR are mL/min/1.73 m^2

4.2.1   Insulin

Patients with diabetes and kidney disease are at increased risk of hypoglycemia due to decreased clearance of some of the medications used to treat diabetes such as insulin, as well as impairment of renal gluconeogenesis from having a lower kidney mass. As the kidney is responsible for about 30–80 % of insulin removal, reduced kidney function is associated with a prolonged insulin half-life and a decrease in insulin requirements as estimated glomerular filtration rate (eGFR) declines [2]. All insulin preparations can be used in patients with CKD, and there is no specified advised reduction in dosing. The insulin type, dose, and administration should be individualized to achieve personal glycemic targets while limiting hypoglycemia. All types of insulin discussed in this chapter are subcutaneous, with the exception of inhaled insulin.

4.2.1.1 Long-Acting Insulin

Long-acting insulin analogs such as U-100 glargine, U-300 glargine, detemir, and degludec are used as basal insulin. U-100 glargine has an onset of action at 2–4 h, with minimal peak and duration of 20–24 h, and is usually dosed once daily. Detemir has an onset of action at 1–3 h, with a small peak at 6–8 h and duration of action of 18–22 h. It is dosed twice daily to give adequate basal coverage in type 1 diabetes; in type 2 diabetes, once-daily dosing can sometimes suffice, depending on the patient. Both U-300 glargine and degludec have a prolonged half-life, and a once-daily dose is virtually always sufficient; no specific dose changes are needed with impaired eGFR with these two types of insulin, other than the general dose reduction often needed for all formulations.

4.2.1.2 Intermediate-Acting Insulin

The only available intermediate-acting insulin is isophane or neutral protamine Hagedorn (NPH). It has an onset of action at 2–4 h, peak concentration at 4–10 h, and duration up to 10–18 h, and is used as a twice-daily basal insulin injection. Its use can be limited by its highly variable absorption, making glargine and detemir preferable choices. However, it is less expensive than glargine and detemir.

4.2.1.3 Short-Acting Insulin

The only short-acting insulin currently available is regular (human or neutral) crystalline insulin, which has an onset of action at about 30 min, peak action at 2–3 h, and duration up to 6 h. Regular crystalline insulin should ideally be given 30 min prior to a meal. It also costs less compared to rapid-acting analogs.

4.2.1.4 Rapid-Acting Insulin

The rapid-acting insulin analogs aspart, lispro, and glulisine are absorbed quickly and are ideal for quick correction of blood sugar or use as prandial insulin. They have an onset of action at about 15 min, peak action at about 60 min, and an average duration of up to 4 h. Rapid-acting insulin can be given up to 15 min before eating and are used in 'basal–bolus' therapy, also known as multiple daily injections (MDI).

Patients with stages 4–5 CKD and those on dialysis may have delayed gastric emptying. In these individuals, giving rapid-acting insulin after a meal may be helpful for matching the insulin peak with the time of the postprandial blood glucose peak.

4.2.1.5 Premixed Insulin Types

Premixed insulin contains a fixed percentage of an intermediate-acting and a rapid- or short-acting insulin. Because they contain a combination of two insulin types, they have two separate peaks. One example is 70/30, which consists of 70 % NPH and 30 % regular insulin. These preparations offer convenience for the patient with twice-daily dosing but offer less flexibility and more restrictions in titration of the insulin. Premixed insulin must be taken at fixed times, and the patient must have consistent meals. 70/30 insulin is sometimes helpful in patients receiving 12-h cycled tube feeds.

4.2.1.6 Different Insulin Concentrations

Insulin is usually U-100 (100 units of insulin/mL). An exception is insulin U-500 (500 units of insulin/mL), which is only available as regular insulin. The high concentration of U-500 alters the properties and pharmacokinetics of regular insulin, leading to a similar onset of action as U-100 (approximately 30 min) but with a peak at 4–8 h and duration of 14–15 h. It can be given up to 30 min prior to meals and is typically given two to three times daily, without the use of any separate basal insulin [3]. U-500 regular insulin is generally used in patients who are severely insulin resistant and can be given as a sub-cutaneous injection or in a pump.

There are other newly available concentrations of other types of insulin, including U-300 glargine, U-200 degludec, and U-200 lispro. These are useful in patients who have elevated insulin resistance and/or who use large amounts of insulin daily. We believe no additional special precautions are needed with these types of insulin, but note U-300 glargine has not been tested in individuals with renal impairment.

4.2.1.7 Inhaled Insulin

Inhaled insulin was approved for use in the United States in 2014. It is a rapid-acting insulin for use as a prandial insulin in adults with type 1 and type 2 diabetes. Its onset of action is at about 12–15 min, peak at 30 min, and duration of action is 3 h. It carries a risk of pulmonary complications and should be avoided in individuals with chronic lung disease. It has not been studied in renal impairment, and it is recommended to adjust dosing to suit the patient's individual needs, as with the use of any type of insulin in a patient with nephropathy.

4.2.2   Oral Medications

4.2.2.1 Metformin

Metformin increases insulin sensitivity and decreases hepatic gluconeogenesis; it does not cause hypoglycemia and can lead to weight loss in some patients. It reduces blood glucose (HbA1c) by 1.0–2.0 % [4]. The most common side effects are diarrhea, bloating, and cramping. Vitamin B12 deficiency has been reported with extended use.

The Food and Drug Administration (FDA) in the United States recently revised its recommendations for metformin so that now it can be used with caution down to an eGFR of 30 mL/min/1.73 m^2. Because metformin is cleared renally, this recommendation is in place to reduce the risk of lactic acidosis in those with even modest renal impairment [5]. The overall incidence of lactic acidosis with metformin use, however, is rare. A Cochrane database review of 347 prospective trials and observational cohort studies showed no cases of fatal or nonfatal lactic acidosis in 70,490 patient-years of metformin users or in 55,451 patient-years of users of other antihyperglycemic agents [6].

Given the differences in translation of creatinine into creatinine clearance based on age, weight, and race, it is reasonable to consider adopting an eGFR-based guideline rather than one based on creatinine alone. Metformin can be used without dose reduction with an eGFR >60 mL/min/1.73 m^2. If the eGFR is ≥45–59 mL/min/1.73 m^2, it is prudent to continue the use of metformin but take caution with dosing and assess renal function every 3–6 months, if possible. If the patient's eGFR is ≥30–44 mL/min/1.73 m^2, again use caution with dosing (e.g., limiting its dose to a maximum of 1000 mg daily or using a 50 % dose reduction), assess renal function every 3 months, and avoid newly initiating metformin in patients with this level of CKD. Metformin should be avoided in patients with an eGFR <30 mL/min/1.73 m^2. It is recommended that metformin is stopped in the presence of situations that are associated with hypoxia or an acute decline in kidney function such as sepsis/shock, hypotension, acute myocardial infarction, and use of radiographic contrast or other nephrotoxic agents [7, 8]. This approach has been accepted by various societies including Kidney Disease: Improving Global Outcomes (KDIGO) and confirmed in additional studies [9–11].

4.2.2.2 Sulfonylureas

Sulfonylureas bind to the sulfonylurea receptor on the pancreatic β-cells and lead to increased insulin secretion. They can cause hypoglycemia and weight gain. The second-generation sulfonylureas — glipizide, glimepiride, glyburide, and gliclazide (the latter is only available in Taiwan) — are commonly prescribed and typically decrease HbA1c by 1–2 % [4].

Sulfonylureas and their metabolites are renally cleared, leading to an increased risk of hypoglycemia as eGFR declines. With an eGFR <60 mL/min/1.73 m², hypoglycemia is greatly increased with glyburide and glimepiride, due to the presence of metabolites cleared in part by the kidneys [12]. Glyburide should be avoided with an eGFR <60 mL/min/1.73 m². Glimepiride should be used with caution if the eGFR is <60 mL/min/1.73 m², and not used with an eGFR <30 mL/min/1.73 m² [12]. Less than 10 % of glipizide is cleared renally, but it should still be used with caution with an eGFR <30 mL/min/1.73 m² due to the risk of hypoglycemia.

4.2.2.3   Glinides

Nateglinide and repaglinide, like sulfonylureas, increase insulin secretion by closing a sulfonylurea receptor/adenosine triphosphate (ATP)-dependent potassium channel on the pancreatic β-cells. They have a shorter half-life compared to the sulfonylureas. They result in a quick release of insulin and should be taken immediately prior to meals. They also can cause hypoglycemia.

The active metabolite of nateglinide accumulates in CKD, and thus, it should not be used in patients with an eGFR <60 mL/min/1.73 m². However, the active metabolite is cleared by hemodialysis, and patients on dialysis can use nateglinide. Conversely, repaglinide appears to be safe for use in individuals with CKD. However, it is reasonable to exercise caution in those with more severe renal dysfunction, such as an eGFR <30 mL/min/1.73 m², and start at the lowest dose (0.5 mg), with a slow up-titration.

4.2.2.4   Thiazolidinediones

Thiazolidinediones (TZDs) such as pioglitazone and rosiglitazone increase insulin sensitivity by acting as peroxisome proliferator-activated receptor (PPAR)-γ agonists. They do not cause hypoglycemia and lower HbA1c by approximately 0.5–1.4 % [4]. They are metabolized by the liver and can be used in CKD. However, fluid retention is a major limiting side effect, and they should not be used in advanced heart failure. This also makes their use in CKD limiting, particularly patients with nephrotic syndrome. TZDs have been linked with increased fracture rates and bone loss; thus, use in patients with underlying bone disease (such as renal osteodystrophy) needs to be carefully considered. No dose adjustment is needed in patients with CKD.

In September 2010, the FDA restricted the use of rosiglitazone based on studies linking it to increased cardiovascular events. After further review, these restrictions were lifted in 2014. An association between pioglitazone and bladder cancer has been raised, but further analysis and investigation into the data show that this association is not clearly supported [13]. A pooled multi-population analysis also showed no association between TZDs and bladder cancer [14].

4.2.2.5 Alpha-Glucosidase Inhibitors

Alpha-glucosidase inhibitors (e.g., acarbose, miglitol) decrease the breakdown of oligo- and disaccharides in the small intestine, slowing ingestion of carbohydrates and delaying absorption of glucose after a meal. The major side effects are bloating, flatulence, and abdominal cramping. They lower HbA1c by 0.5–0.8 % and usually do not lead to any changes in weight [4].

Acarbose is minimally absorbed orally with only <2 % of the drug and active metabolites present in the urine. With reduced renal function, serum levels of acarbose and metabolites are significantly higher. Miglitol has greater systemic absorption, with >95 % renal excretion. It is recommended that the use of miglitol should be avoided if a patient has an eGFR of <25 mL/min/1.73 m^2. Additionally, alpha-glucosidase inhibitors have not yet been studied long-term in patients with creatinine >2 mg/dL, and so their use should be avoided in these patients.

4.2.2.6 Dipeptidyl Peptidase-4 Inhibitors

Dipeptidyl peptidase-4 (DPP-4) inhibitors decrease the breakdown of incretin hormones such as glucagon-like peptide-1 (GLP-1) and include sitagliptin, saxagliptin, linagliptin, and alogliptin. This class of medication is weight neutral and decreases HbA1c by 0.5–0.8 % [4].

Approximately 80 % of sitagliptin is cleared by the kidneys. For patients with an eGFR of $\geq$30 to <50 mL/min/1.73 m^2, 50 mg once daily should be used; with an eGFR <30 mL/min/1.73 m^2, a dose of 25 mg once daily is advised. Saxagliptin also requires a dose reduction (to 2.5 mg daily) when given to patients with an eGFR $\leq$ 50 mL/min/1.73 m^2 to 2.5 mg; otherwise, the standard dose of 2.5–5.0 mg daily can be used with an eGFR >50 mL/min/1.73 m^2. Only a small amount of linagliptin is cleared renally; thus, no dose adjustment is needed with a reduced GFR. Alogliptin also necessitates a dose reduction, from the baseline dose of 25 mg daily to 12.5 mg daily with an eGFR <60 mL/min/1.73 m^2 and then to 6.25 mg daily in patients with an eGFR <30 mL/min/1.73 m^2.

4.2.2.7 Sodium–Glucose Cotransporter 2 Inhibitors

Sodium-glucose cotransporter 2 (SGLT2) inhibitors (e.g., canagliflozin, dapagliflozin, empagliflozin) reduce glucose absorption in the kidneys, leading to an increase in glucose excretion in the urine and a reduction in HbA1c of about 0.9–1.0 % [15]. The increase in urine glucose can result in a weight loss of up to 5 kg/year. Because of an increase in adverse events related to intravascular volume contraction, no more than 100 mg once daily of canagliflozin should be used in patients with an eGFR of 45 mL to <60 mL/min/1.73 m^2. Its use should be avoided if the patient's eGFR is <45 mL/min/1.73 m^2 because of an increase in risk of adverse events, as well as reduced efficacy. Dapagliflozin is not approved for use if eGFR is < 60 mL/min/1.73 m^2; empagliflozin can be used down to an eGFR of 45 mL/min/1.73 m^2. There have been rare cases of ketoacidosis associated with use of SGLT2 inhibitors in patients who require insulin for type 1 or type 2 diabetes.

4.2.2.8 Other Oral Medications

Bromocriptine (dopamine receptor agonist) has not been adequately studied in CKD. Colesevelam (bile acid sequestrant) shows no difference in efficacy or safety in those with an eGFR <50 mL/min/1.73 m^2, but data are limited, as it has not been adequately studied in more advanced CKD.

4.2.3   Other Subcutaneous Medications

4.2.3.1 Glucagon-Like Peptide-1 Receptor Agonists

Exenatide (regular and extended-release) and liraglutide are injectable medications that mimic gut hormones called incretins, leading to insulin release, decreased glucagon secretion, and delayed gastric emptying. They are FDA approved for use with metformin and/or sulfonylureas; exenatide, liraglutide, and albiglutide are also approved for use with basal but not prandial insulin. They contribute to central satiety leading to a reduction in appetite and often weight loss. The average expected HbA1c decrease is 0.5–1.0 % [4]. These agents have been associated with pancreatitis, but epidemiologic studies have not supported an increased risk. Nausea is a common side effect that can limit its use. In addition, liraglutide has been associated with the development of thyroid C-cell tumors in animal studies and thus should not be given to patients with or at risk for medullary thyroid cancer. Exenatide is given twice daily, and liraglutide is given once daily; exenatide extended-release is dosed once weekly. Albiglutide and dulaglutide are other GLP-1 receptor agonists that can also be dosed once weekly.

Clearance of exenatide decreases with declines in eGFR [16]. The FDA reported cases of acute renal failure associated with exenatide use and recommends it be used with caution in those with an eGFR of 30–50 mL/min/1.73 m^2 and not be used if the eGFR is <30 mL/min/1.73 m^2. Liraglutide is not metabolized primarily by the kidney; no dose adjustment is indicated in those with renal impairment, including end-stage renal disease (ESRD), although data in this population are limited [17]. The manufacturer has reported cases of renal failure and worsening of chronic renal impairment with use and advises caution with initiating or increasing the dose in those with nephropathy. No dosage restrictions are needed for albiglutide or dulaglutide with decreasing eGFR.

4.2.3.2 Amylin Analog

Amylin is secreted along with insulin by pancreatic β-cells, and levels are low in patients with diabetes. Pramlintide is an injectable amylin analog taken with meals as an adjunct to insulin therapy in type 1 and type 2 diabetes. It reduces HbA1c by 0.5–1.0 % [4]. No dose adjustment appears necessary for CKD; it has not been studied in ESRD.

4.3 Glycemic Control in Chronic Kidney Disease

4.3.1 Strategy for Glycemic Control and Other Risk Factors

The ideal medication regimen is based on the specific needs of the patient and physician experience and should be individualized, especially as renal function changes. An individual with type 1 diabetes needs insulin, and there are multiple ways insulin can be administered. A wide range of therapies can be applied to those with type 2 diabetes.

4.3.1.1 Type 1 Diabetes Mellitus

The ideal insulin regimen in type 1 diabetes reproduces physiologic insulin secretion by the pancreas, most often accomplished by the use of a basal insulin and pre-meal injections of rapid-acting insulin. An even closer approximation of physiologic insulin secretion is through the use of an insulin pump that delivers a continuous subcutaneous infusion of insulin (CSII). A rapid-acting analog is infused via the pump and serves as the basal, bolus, and correction insulin. Insulin pumps can be used at all stages of CKD. Insulin pumps require vigilance on the part of the patient, and their use should be overseen by endocrinologists and experienced diabetes educators.

4.3.1.2 Type 2 Diabetes Mellitus

Multiple options and combinations of therapies are available for patients with type 2 diabetes. Oral medications are an ideal starting point. Metformin is a first-line agent because it does not cause hypoglycemia, is associated with weight loss, and is inexpensive. It can cause gastrointestinal symptoms, and the dose should be increased slowly. Dosing in CKD is discussed above. The sulfonylureas are also a reasonable choice as they are inexpensive and are effective, but they do cause hypoglycemia. In CKD, glipizide or gliclazide is preferable. DPP-4 inhibitors can be safely used at the appropriate dose in CKD, though the reduction in HbA1c and hyperglycemia is modest with an average reduction in HbA1c between 0.5 and 1.0 %. Pioglitazone can be considered, though fluid retention, weight gain, and a small lowering of the HbA1c make it a less optimal choice. SGLT2 inhibitors are reasonable choices if kidney function allows use. GLP-1 receptor agonists can be added to oral agents such as sulfonylureas, but they should not be used concurrently with DPP-4 inhibitors; in CKD, liraglutide is preferred to exenatide, and dulaglutide and albiglutide can also be used. The injection may not be desirable, but the potential for reduction in hyperglycemia, weight loss, and option for weekly dosing can be appealing. They can also be used as single agents.

In patients with uncontrolled HbA1c levels, high levels of insulin resistance, or progressive β-cell failure, insulin should be introduced. A basal insulin such as once-daily glargine, detemir, degludec, or twice-daily NPH is initiated first. A starting dose of 10–15 units can be used, with further escalation based on blood sugars. Some patients may achieve goal glucose control with the combination of basal insulin and oral agents. Basal insulin may also be combined with the GLP-1 receptor agonists exenatide, liraglutide, and albiglutide. If the goal glycemic control cannot be obtained with basal insulin, then a rapid-acting insulin should be started.

4.3.2   Glycemic Goal Targeting

In general, the recommended target HbA1c for diabetes control by the American Diabetes Association (ADA) has been less than or around 7 % [18]. The ADA advises higher (<8 %) or stricter (<6.5 %) HbA1c goals for certain populations [18]. The American Association of Clinical Endocrinologists (AACE) suggests a goal HbA1c of ≤6.5 % in healthy patients who are at low risk for hypoglycemia but also acknowledges the goals need to be individualized [19]. The 2007 Kidney Disease Outcomes Quality Initiative (KDOQI) guidelines for diabetes and CKD endorse a target HbA1c of <7.0 % [20], but their updated 2012 guidelines instead recommend an HbA1c of ~7.0 % [21].

In type 1 diabetes, a number of studies show that the development of microalbuminuria is associated with poorer glycemic control. In the Diabetes Control and Complications Trial (DCCT), intensive therapy in patients with type 1 diabetes (mean HbA1c 9.1 % vs. 7.2 %) reduced the occurrence of microalbuminuria and risk reduction in progression to clinical albuminuria [22, 23]. In patients with type 2 diabetes, the Kumamoto study, UK Prospective Diabetes Study (UKPDS), and Veterans Affairs Cooperative studies showed reduction of new onset nephropathy and progression of nephropathy with intensive glycemic control [24–26].

The ACCORD study showed higher risk of hypoglycemia and mortality in patients with type 2 diabetes treated with intensive glucose control (mean HbA1c 6.4 % vs. 7.5 %), without any risk reduction on cardiovascular disease (CVD). The increased mortality could not be attributed to hypoglycemia [27]. In the ADVANCE trial, more intensive glycemic control (HbA1c 6.5 % vs. 7.3 %) showed no reduction in CVD. However, the intensive group had a 21 % reduction in nephropathy [28].

The Veteran's Affairs Diabetes Trial (VADT) study (intensive group with HbA1c 6.9 % vs. 8.4 %) also showed no benefit on CVD risk with stricter glucose control [29].

The data clearly show that lowering HbA1c leads to benefit in regard to nephropathy. Benefits in HbA1c reduction are also seen on rates of retinopathy and neuropathy. However, the effect of lowering HbA1c is much less in regards to macrovascular disease. Overall, it is reasonable that a target HbA1c ~7.0 % offers an optimal risk to benefit ratio rather than a target that is much lower.

4.3.3   Adjusting the Glycemic Goal in Chronic Kidney Disease

Lower HbA1c levels are associated with higher risks of hypoglycemia so the HbA1c target should be individualized. Consequences of hypoglycemia, such as injury, myocardial infarction, seizure, stroke, or death, are highest in those who are frail and elderly, with erratic eating habits, on insulin and sulfonylureas, and with CKD. Higher HbA1c targets should be considered for those with shortened life expectancies, a known history of severe hypoglycemia or hypoglycemia unawareness, CKD, and children.

The Controversies Conference on DKD held by KDIGO addressed a number of issues surrounding DKD, including appropriate glycemic control targets [11]. There are insufficient data and trials regarding the ideal glucose target in patients with CKD stage 3 or worse. Patients with ESRD and diabetes benefit from maintaining their HbA1c between 7 and 8 %, as HbA1c levels above 8 % or below 7 % carry increased risks of all-cause and cardiovascular death.

4.4   Other Risk Factors

The combination of diabetes and CKD is potent in regard to cardiovascular disease risk. Lifestyle changes to control weight, improve nutrition, and modify dietary intake and exercise should be encouraged. Blood pressure control and dyslipidemia should be addressed as well.

4.5   Conclusion

The management of patients with diabetes and nephropathy necessitates attention to several aspects of care. Importantly, glycemic control should be optimized for the patient, attaining the necessary control to reduce complications but done in a safe, monitored manner and knowing which medication can be used safely. Treatment of diabetes and nephropathy necessitates a multifactorial approach through the use of a diabetologist, nephrologist, and diabetes educator.

References

1. American Diabetes Association (ADA). Microvascular complications and foot care. Sec. 9. Standards of Medical Care in Diabetes – 2015. Diabetes Care. 2016;39:S72–80.
2. Rabkin R, Ryan MP, Duckworth WC. The renal metabolism of insulin. Diabetologia. 1984;27:351–7.
3. de la Pena A, Riddle M, Morrow LA, Jiang HH, Linnebjerg H, Scott A, et al. Pharmacokinetics and pharmacodynamics of high-dose human regular U-500 insulin versus human regular U-100 insulin in healthy obese subjects. Diabetes Care. 2011;34: 2496–501.
4. Nathan DM, Buse JB, Davidson MB, Ferrannini E, Holman RR, Sherwin R, et al. Medical management of hyperglycemia in type 2 diabetes: a consensus algorithm for the initiation and adjustment of therapy: a consensus statement of the American Diabetes Association and the European Association for the Study of Diabetes. Diabetes Care. 2009;32:193–203.
5. Sambol NC, Chiang J, Lin ET, Goodman AM, Liu CY, Benet LZ, Cogan MG. Kidney function and age are both predictors of pharmacokinetics of metformin. J Clin Pharm. 1995;35:1094–102.
6. Salpeter SR, Greyber E, Pasternak GA, Salpeter EE. Risk of fatal and nonfatal lactic acidosis with metformin use in type 2 diabetes mellitus. Cochrane Database Syst Rev. 2010;(2): CD002967.
7. Inzucchi SE, Lipska KJ, Mayo H, Bailey CJ, McGuire DK. Metformin in patients with type 2 diabetes and kidney disease: a systematic review. JAMA. 2014;312:2668–75.

8. Herrington WG, Levy JB. Metformin: effective and safe in renal disease? Int Urol Nephrol. 2008;40:411–7.
9. Eppenga WL, Lalmohamed A, Geerts AF, Derijks HJ, Wensing M, Egberts A, et al. Risk of lactic acidosis or elevated lactate concentrations in metformin users with renal impairment: a population-based cohort study. Diabetes Care. 2014;37:2218–24.
10. Richy FF, Sabido-Espin M, Guedes S, Corvino FA, Gottwald-Hostalek U. Incidence of lactic acidosis in patients with type 2 diabetes with and without renal impairment treated with metformin: a retrospective cohort study. Diabetes Care. 2014;37:2291–5.
11. Molitch ME, Adler AI, Flyvbjerg A, Nelson RG, So WY, Wanner C, et al. Diabetic kidney disease: a clinical update from Kidney Disease: Improving Global Outcomes. Kidney Int. 2014;87:20–30.
12. Holstein A, Plaschke A, Hammer C, Ptak M, Kuhn J, Kratzsch C, et al. Hormonal counterregulation and consecutive glimepiride serum concentrations during severe hypoglycaemia associated with glimepiride therapy. Eur J Clin Pharm. 2003;59:747–54.
13. Ryder RE. Pioglitazone has a dubious bladder cancer risk but an undoubted cardiovascular benefit. Diabetic Med. 2015;32:305–13.
14. Levin D, Bell S, Sund R, Hartikainen SA, Tuomilehto J, Pukkala E, et al. Pioglitazone and bladder cancer risk: a multipopulation pooled, cumulative exposure analysis. Diabetologia. 2015;58:493–504.
15. Kalra S. Sodium glucose co-transporter-2 (SGLT2) inhibitors: a review of their basic and clinical pharmacology. Diabetes Ther. 2014;5:355–66.
16. Linnebjerg H, Kothare PA, Park S, Mace K, Reddy S, Mitchell M, et al. Effect of renal impairment on the pharmacokinetics of exenatide. Br J Clin Pharmacol. 2007;64:317–27.
17. Davidson JA, Brett J, Falahati A, Scott D. Mild renal impairment and the efficacy and safety of liraglutide. Endocr Pract. 2011;17:345–55.
18. American Diabetes Association (ADA). Glycemic targets. Sec. 5. Standards of Medical Care in Diabetes – 2015. Diabetes Care. 2016;39:S39–46.
19. Garber AJ, Abrahamson MJ, Barzilay JI, Blonde L, Bloomgarden ZT, Bush MA, et al. American Association of Clinical Endocrinologists (AACE) comprehensive diabetes management algorithm 2013. Endocrin Pract. 2013;19:327–36.

20. Kidney Disease Outcomes Quality Initiative (KDOQI). KDOQI Clinical Practice Guidelines and Clinical Practice Recommendations for Diabetes and Chronic Kidney Disease. Am J Kidney Dis. 2007;49:S12–154.

21. Kidney Disease Outcomes Quality Initiative (KDOQI). KDOQI Clinical Practice Guideline for Diabetes and CKD: 2012 Update. Am J Kidney Dis. 2012;60:850–86.

22. Diabetes Control and Complications Trial Research Group (DCCT). The effect of intensive treatment of diabetes on the development and progression of long-term complications in insulin-dependent diabetes mellitus. The Diabetes Control and Complications Trial Research Group. N Engl J Med. 1993;329:977–86.

23. Diabetes Control and Complications Trial Research (DCCT). Effect of intensive therapy on the development and progression of diabetic nephropathy in the Diabetes Control and Complications Trial. Kidney Int. 1995;47:1703–20.

24. Levin SR, Coburn JW, Abraira C, Henderson WG, Colwell JA, Emanuele NV, et al. Effect of intensive glycemic control on microalbuminuria in type 2 diabetes. Veterans Affairs Cooperative Study on Glycemic Control and Complications in Type 2 Diabetes Feasibility Trial Investigators. Diabetes Care. 2000;23:1478–85.

25. Ohkubo Y, Kishikawa H, Araki E, Miyata T, Isami S, Motoyoshi S, et al. Intensive insulin therapy prevents the progression of diabetic microvascular complications in Japanese patients with non-insulin-dependent diabetes mellitus: a randomized prospective 6-year study. Diabetes Res Clin Pract. 1995;28:103–17.

26. UK Prospective Diabetes Study (UKPDS) Group. Intensive blood-glucose control with sulphonylureas or insulin compared with conventional treatment and risk of complications in patients with type 2 diabetes (UKPDS 33). Lancet. 1998;352:837–53.

27. Gerstein HC, Miller ME, Byington RP, Goff Jr DC, Bigger JT, Buse JB, et al. Effects of intensive glucose lowering in type 2 diabetes. N Engl J Med. 2008;358:2545–59.

28. Patel A, MacMahon S, Chalmers J, Neal B, Billot L, Woodward M, et al. Intensive blood glucose control and vascular outcomes in patients with type 2 diabetes. N Engl J Med. 2008;358:2560–72.

29. Duckworth W, Abraira C, Moritz T, Reda D, Emanuele N, Reaven PD, et al. Glucose control and vascular complications in veterans with type 2 diabetes. N Engl J Med. 2009;360:129–39.

Chapter 5
Management of Overt Diabetic Kidney Disease and Uremia

Guntram Schernthaner and Friedrich C. Prischl

5.1   Introduction

Once long-standing diabetes has involved the kidneys, the process of ongoing damage to predominantly glomerular structures cannot be stopped by currently available therapeutic interventions. Kidney damage is considered to be clinically 'silent' (lacking obvious symptoms) and may present in two forms. Most commonly, proteinuria, starting as microalbuminuria, is the leading presentation. However, in approximately one in every seven patients, a reduction in estimated glomerular filtration (eGFR), without any type of albuminuria, is the first sign of kidney involvement in diabetes [1].

Therefore, various authors have started using the term diabetic kidney disease (DKD), instead of diabetic nephropathy (DN), as DN is commonly associated with patients presenting with albuminuria only. In the United Kingdom Prospective Diabetes Study (UKPDS), approximately 15 % of patients in the study had a reduced eGFR at the time of detection of albuminuria [1]. Additionally, an analysis found a prevalence of normoalbuminuric DKD of 9.7 % (i.e., one in ten patients with diabetes) [2]. As a result, the American Diabetes Association (ADA) used DKD (not DN) in its most recent position statement on medical care in diabetes [3].

G.L. Bakris et al., *Managing Diabetic Nephropathies in Clinical Practice*, DOI 10.1007/978-3-319-08873-0_5,
© Springer International Publishing Switzerland 2017

5.2   Epidemiology

A recent analysis revealed an estimated diabetes prevalence of 12–14 % among adults in the United States, increasing between the periods of 1988–1994 and 2011–2012 in the overall population and in all subgroups evaluated [4]. In the age group ≥65 years, this amounts to more than 20 %. Accordingly, an analysis from the National Health and Nutrition Examination Survey (NHANES) indicates that the incidence and prevalence of diabetes-related complications such as DKD are expected to rise as well [4].

Using the NHANES database, Bailey et al. showed a dramatically high prevalence of DKD in patients with type 2 diabetes: 43.5 %, with half of them being ≥65 years of age [5]. The DKD categorization was based on the Kidney Disease Improving Global Outcomes (KDIGO) classification of either reduced eGFR and/or urinary albumin excretion (UAE) [6]. As shown in Fig 5.1, in stages 3, 4, and 5, an increase in prevalence emerges over time, whereas in stages 1 and 2, no such trend is seen [4]. However, the prevalence of DKD seems to differ according to country. Over a period of 20 years, 32 studies from 16 countries revealed a prevalence ranging from 11 to 83 % of patients with diabetes [7].

5.2.1   Incidence of Diabetic Kidney Disease-Related End-Stage Renal Disease

With regard to end-stage renal disease (ESRD) in developed countries, DKD is the leading cause of ESRD requiring renal replacement therapy (RRT) [8]. According to the United States Renal Data System (USRDS) 2014 Annual Data Report (referring to data from 2012), the incidence of ESRD requiring RRT was 114,813 patients, with 44 % due to DKD [9]. A registry report from Japan revealed a nearly identical relative incidence, with 44.2 % of the patients with ESRD caused by diabetes [10].

In absolute numbers, the incidence of DKD-related ESRD had risen dramatically since 1980 but declined slightly from 2010 to 2012. With regard to the incidence rate of DKD-related ESRD per million per year, the incidence 'plateau' was reached in 2000. This amounts to 353 per million/year in 2012 (according to the most recent available data). Interestingly, ESRD incidence has declined in the past decade. This is in line with results from a nationwide analysis on DKD with ESRD in Austria from 1965 to 2013 showing that both absolute numbers, as well as adjusted incidence, have been declining since 2006 [11]. A recent report from the

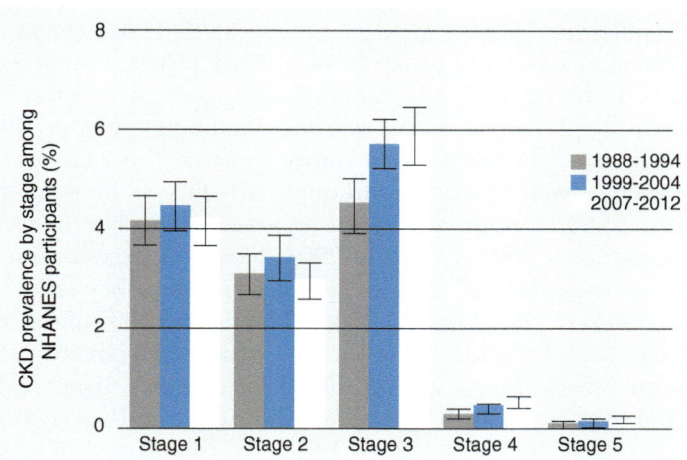

FIGURE 5.1 Prevalence of chronic kidney disease by stage among National Health and Nutrition Examination Survey (NHANES) participants, 1988–2012. Time periods included 1988–1994, 1999–2004, and 2007–2012. In participants aged 20 years and older. Stage 1: eGFR $\geq$90 mL/min/1.73 m^2 and ACR $\geq$ 30 mg/g; stage 2: eGFR 60–89 mL/min/1.73 m^2 and ACR $\geq$30 mg/g; stage 3: eGFR 30–59 mL/min/1.73 m^2; stage 4: eGFR 15–29 mL/min/1.73 m^2; stage 5: eGFR <15 mL/min/1.73 m^2. Whisker lines indicate 95 % confidence intervals. *CKD* chronic kidney disease (Reproduced with permission from NHANES [4] ©United States Renal Data System)

European Renal Association–European Dialysis and Transplant Association Registry in Europe using data from 1998 to 2011 confirmed a decline of the adjusted annual incidence of 2.2 % in the overall ESRD population during 2008–2011, mainly derived from patients with DKD. The annual percentage change of incidence per million population (PMP), in patients with type 1 and type 2 diabetes was −2.4 % (95 % CI, −3.8 to −0.8) from 2007 to 2011 [12].

5.2.2   Prevalence of Diabetic Kidney Disease-Related End-Stage Renal Disease

Prevalence is highly variable with regard to different populations [11–14]. It may be as low as 78.0 PMP (Iceland, Romania), but may go up to 743.1 PMP (United States) or 902 PMP (Japan). Prevalence has appeared to increase steadily due to various reasons, including demographic changes, and decreased mortality from cardiovascular and other causes of death. Although still higher than in the nondiabetic population, in representative US cohorts assessed in 1997–1998 and 2003–2004, the excess annual cardiovascular and the all-cause death rate associated with diabetes declined from 5.8 to 2.3 deaths per 1000 and from 10.8 to 6.1 deaths per 1000 at risk, respectively [15]. Conversely, the prevalence of DKD increased from 2.2 % in 1988–1994 to 3.3 % in 2005–2008 [16], and survival of patients with DKD-related ESRD has improved in some countries (e.g., Austria) [11].

5.3   Onset of Overt Diabetic Kidney Disease

Patients with overt DKD typically have a history of diabetes of 5 years or more. Depending on the beginning of the disease, patients with type 1 diabetes are markedly younger than type 2 patients. The latter usually develop ESRD in their mid-fifties to mid-sixties. According to a small but carefully conducted study, both type 1 and type 2 patients take an average of 77–81 months from the stage of producing macroproteinuria with near-normal renal function to developing ESRD [17].

When a patient with diabetes-related kidney involvement is first examined, it must be determined whether their kidney disease is due to DKD or other forms of kidney disease (e.g., glomerulonephritis). Carefully taking a family history should be done to rule out hereditary disease such as polycystic kidney disease and Alport syndrome to give an example.

Laboratory analyses at diagnosis should include serum creatinine, blood urea nitrogen, eGFR, sodium, potassium, calcium, phosphate, blood gas analysis, hematocrit, urine dipstick analysis, urine microalbuminuria, microscopic examination of urine, and albumin/creatinine ratio in urine. In special cases, a 24-h urine collection with analysis of creatinine clearance and quantification of proteinuria may be necessary. For all patients suspected of developing DKD, regular follow-up laboratory examinations should include analysis of serum creatinine, eGFR, sodium, potassium, calcium, phosphate, and urine albumin/creatinine ratio. Blood and urine tests may have to be extended according to the stage of kidney dysfunction, slope of progression, or presence of comorbid conditions. If a kidney transplantation is strived for, special protocols on preoperative laboratory tests will be determined by individual transplant centers.

In case of anemia, renal anemia (responsive to erythropoiesis-stimulating agents) has to be suspected, but other causes have to be ruled out (e.g., occult gastrointestinal bleeding). Iron deficiency should be considered (as determined by measurement of iron, ferritin, transferrin, transferrin saturation, and percentage of hypochromic red cells). Rarely, vitamin B12/folate deficiency may be indicated by macrocytic anemia. Bone mineral disorders in chronic kidney disease (CKD; eGFR <60 mL/min) should also be ruled out. This can be determined by measuring parathyroid hormone and vitamin D levels.

Hypertension is present in up to 85 % of patients with DN/DKD, depending on the duration and stage (e.g., higher in more progressive cases). Eventually, coronary artery disease and other manifestations of arterial disease may develop. Other signs of microangiopathy (e.g., diabetic retinopathy) are present, but often are not diagnosed at the first presentation of DKD. With presence of overt proteinuria (above 1 g in 24 h), edema may be present, predominantly of the eyelids, ankle, and legs. With disease that is more progressive, pleural effusions or even ascites may be present. In more pronounced cases, patients may report dyspnea on exertion. Nycturia is also common.

Some patients may first present to their doctors already at stage 5 in pre-uremia or uremia. In these cases, dyspnea (New York Heart Association [NYHA] classifications II to IV), edema, anasarca, and/or skin discoloration may be the predominant signs. Further, angina, neurologic symptoms (i.e., dizziness, confusion, peripheral neuropathy, even coma), loss of appetite, nausea, vomiting, changes in bowel movements (i.e., reduced texture of stool), and very dry skin with pruritus may also be present.

5.3.1   Differential Diagnosis

A further examination by a nephrologist has to be considered in patients who have signs and symptoms, including the following:

- Proven duration of diabetes of <5 years.
- Signs of microangiopathy elsewhere (e.g., proliferative diabetic retinopathy) are missing.
- Microhematuria with microscopic examination of urine showing acanthocytes (characteristically deformed erythrocytes). Exemption: microhematuria may be present also in diabetic nephropathy when ischemia has acutely led to renal papillary necrosis.
- Red (erythrocyte) casts/leucocyte casts in microscopic examination of urine.
- Rapid onset and increase of albuminuria/proteinuria within days/weeks.

- Rapid increase of serum creatinine.
- Abnormal findings during a kidney ultrasound examination (e.g., marked difference in size of kidneys, hydronephrosis).

Hypertensive or ischemic nephropathy may be present in patients with diabetes. Especially in cases of nephrotic range proteinuria, other kidney diseases such as focal segmental glomerulosclerosis, glomerulonephritis, and kidney involvement due to other systemic diseases (e.g., amyloidosis, multiple myeloma) must be ruled out. In addition, acute injuries such as acute interstitial nephritis have to be considered [18].

5.4   Glycemic Control

5.4.1   Glucose-Lowering Therapeutic Options in Patients with Diabetic Kidney Disease

The armamentarium of therapeutic agents used for the treatment of diabetes has expanded over the past decade. In fact, ten classes of glucose-lowering agents are now available. However, the pharmacokinetic properties of many of these drugs are altered in patients with kidney dysfunction and may require dose adjustment or avoidance in patients on dialysis [19, 20]. When selecting and dosing glucose-lowering drugs, renal function has to be assessed and periodically monitored during treatment to detect changes that may affect drug metabolism and excretion. Whereas patients with mild renal insufficiency can receive most antihyperglycemic treatments without any concern, patients with CKD stage 3a and, in particular, with CKD stages 3b, 4, and 5 often require treatment adjustments according to the degree of renal insufficiency [21]. These adjustments include dose reduction or discontinuation of a drug and, if necessary, initiation of another drug.

Newer drugs that do not increase the risk for hypoglycemia may improve treatment options for patients with type 2 diabetes. For example, because linagliptin has a very low rate of renal excretion (5 %; the majority [80 %] is excreted via the enterohepatic system), it can be used without any dose reduction at all stages of CKD and has been shown to be safe in renal impairment as well as in older patients with type 2 diabetes [22, 23].

Sodium–glucose cotransporter 2 (SGLT2) inhibitors are emerging as new therapies with complementary mechanisms of action that are independent of insulin secretion or action [24]. SGLT2 inhibitors lower plasma glucose by lowering the renal threshold of glucose, leading to increased urinary glucose excretion (UGE) and a mild osmotic diuresis. Several studies have confirmed the efficacy of SGLT2 inhibitors in improving glycemic control with a low risk of hypoglycemia plus several pleiotropic effects, including weight loss, lowering of blood pressure (BP) and an improvement in the metabolic milieu (e.g., triglyceride, uric acid, and high-density lipoprotein [HDL] levels). When ß-cell function is declining, dipeptidyl peptidase-4 (DPP-4) inhibitors are inferior to SGLT2 inhibitors in terms of lowering hemoglobin A1c (HbA1c) and do not cause weight loss or blood pressure lowering [25]. There is increasing evidence that SGLT2 inhibitors may provide renoprotection [26]. This renoprotection may be derived from direct effects such as attenuating diabetes-associated hyperfiltration and tubular hypertrophy, as well as reducing the tubular toxicity of glucose. Indirect effects include improving glycemic control, insulin sensitivity, weight control (due to modest reductions in body weight), and blood pressure control (due to the natriuretic effect and weight loss and lowering uric acid levels). It has been assumed that these beneficial effects may not be present in patients with established renal impairment, as the magnitude of glucose excretion and HbA1c reduction induced by SGLT2 inhibitors is dependent upon the filtered glucose load and is maximal in diabetic subjects with a normal glomerular filtration rate.

Recently, impressive cardioprotection was documented for empagliflozin, an SGLT2 inhibitor, when it was given to patients with diabetes, and established cardiovascular disease (CVD) in the EMPA-REG Outcome study [27]. Although the patients were well treated (50 % of the patients received insulin, 75 % metformin, 77 % statins, 80 % angiotensin-converting enzyme [ACE]/angiotensin receptor blockers [ARB], and 90 % antiplatelet agents), all-cause mortality and CV mortality were reduced by 32 % and 38 %, respectively, in patients randomized to empagliflozin when compared to placebo (hazard ratio [HR] 0.86; 95 % CI, 0.74–0.99; $P = 0.04$ for superiority) [28]. Surprisingly, renoprotection was observed in patients with eGFR < 60 mL/min randomized to empagliflozin, as shown by reductions in creatinine doubling, progression to ESRD, and renal death (HR 0.54; 95 % CI, 0.40–0.75; $P = 0.0002$) [28]. In fact, new-onset or worsening kidney disease was reduced by 39 %, macroalbuminuria by 38 %, doubling of serum creatinine by 44 %, and incidence of ESRD by 55 %. Importantly, CVD outcomes were not worse in patients with comorbid CVD and CKD, compared to those without CKD [28]. It is important to mention that the majority of patients had impaired kidney function at baseline: 52.2 % were stage 2, 17.8 % were stage 3a, and 7.7 % were stage 3b; all patients with CKD stages 4 and 5 were excluded from the EMPA-REG Outcome study [27].

Metformin is widely viewed as the best initial pharmacological option to lower glucose concentration in patients with type 2 diabetes. Metformin is also widely used in all combination therapies. However, this drug is contraindicated in many individuals with impaired kidney function because of concerns of lactic acidosis. Although metformin is cleared renally, drug levels generally remain within the therapeutic range, and lactate concentrations are not substantially increased when used in patients with mild to moderate CKD (eGFR 30–60 mL/min per 1.73 m^2). The overall incidence of lactic acidosis in metformin users varies across studies from approximately 3–10 per 100,000 person-years and is generally indistinguishable from the background rate in the overall population with diabetes. A recent review [29] summarized that the use of metformin in patients with mild to moderate renal impairment is associated with a decrease in CV mortality and all-cause mortality, but metformin must be stopped in patients with CKD stage 5, because in these patients, an increased all-cause mortality was recently reported [30]. Detailed dose recommendations for all available glucose-lowering drugs in CKD as provided in various labels in the United States, EU, and Canada have been summarized in a recent review [31].

5.4.2   Glycemic Control for Patients Undergoing Hemodialysis

It is well known that the 5-year survival rate is much lower in diabetic versus nondiabetic patients undergoing hemodialysis (HD) [23]. During the last 15 years, several observational studies were published indicating that the survival of diabetic patients on HD is influenced by the glycemic control. For example, Morioka et al. evaluated the impact of glycemic control on survival in 150 diabetic subjects with ESRD starting HD treatment. During the short follow-up period of 2.8 years, 76 % of the patients died; however, in those with good control (HbA1c <7.5 %), mortality was lower than in those with poor glycemic control (HbA1c ≥7.5 %) [32]. Oomichi et al. found in a 7-year observational study of 114 patients with diabetes on HD that mortality was similar in patients with HbA1c <6.5 % and fair glycemic control (HbA1c >6.5 % to <8.0 %), but mortality was significantly higher (HR 2.89; $P = 0.01$) in those with poor glycemic control (HbA1c >8.0 %) [33]. Hayashino et al. analyzed mortality in the large Japanese Dialysis Outcomes and Practice Pattern Study on 1569 HD patients with diabetes and 3342 HD patients without diabetes. Mortality was significantly higher in patients with diabetes on HD with an HbA1c in the fifth quintile (HbA1c ≥7.3 %), but was not different in the other four quintiles (HbA1c 5.0–7.2 %) [34]. Kalantar-Zadeh et al. evaluated 23,618 patients with diabetes undergoing HD in the United States and evaluated survival as a function of

HbA1c [35]. They observed that higher HbA1c values were incrementally associated with higher mortality. Compared with patients with HbA1c in the range of 5–6 %, patients with HbA1c >10 % had higher HRs of adjusted all-cause and CV death: 1.41 and 1.73 ($P < 0.001$), respectively [35]. Remarkably, this relationship was only seen in patients without anemia (Hb > 11.0 g/day; $n = 19,316$) and not in patients with anemia or malnutrition. Drechsler et al. investigated the impact of glycemic control on CV outcomes in 1255 patients with diabetes on HD in the German Diabetes and Dialysis Study (4D Study) [36]. During 4 years of follow-up, patients with HbA1c >8.0 % or HbA1c from >6 to <8 % had an increased risk of sudden death (HR 1.85 and 2.26, respectively; $P < 0.003$) compared with patients with HbA1c <6.0 %. In contrast, the risk of myocardial infarction (MI) and all-cause mortality did not differ between the three groups.

A recent meta-analysis of observational studies or randomized controlled trials investigating the association between HbA1c values and mortality risk in patients with diabetes receiving HD confirmed that poor glycemic control is associated with an increased mortality [37]. In total, ten studies (83,684 participants; 9 observational studies and a secondary analysis of a randomized trial) were included. After adjusting for confounding elements, patients with baseline HbA1c levels ≥8.5 % (≥69 mmol/mol) had increased mortality (7 studies; HR 1.14; 95 % CI, 1.09–1.19) when compared with patients with HbA1c levels of 6.5–7.4 % (48–57 mmol/mol). Likewise, patients with a mean HbA1c value ≥8.5 % also had a higher adjusted risk of mortality (6 studies; HR 1.29; 95 % CI, 1.23–1.35). There was a small but nonsignificant increase in mortality associated with mean HbA1c levels ≤5.4 % (≤36 mmol/mol; 6 studies; HR 1.09; 95 % CI, 0.89–1.34) [37].

In the UK, one-third of patients receiving HD have diabetes. Guidelines from organizations representing patients with renal disease and diabetes advocate tight glycemic control in patients with ESRD, despite glucose-lowering trials having excluded these patients. Using the national UK Renal Registry data,

Adler et al. tested whether HbA1c levels were associated with death in adults with diabetes starting HD or peritoneal dialysis [38]. Of 3157 patients observed for a median time of 2.7 years, 1688 died. For patients ≥60 years of age, they found no association between HbA1c and death; among younger patients, relative to those with HbA1c values 6.5–7.4 %, the HR for HbA1c 7.5–8.4 % was 1.2 (95 % CI, 0.9–1.5), and for HbA1c >8.5 %, HR was 1.5 (95 % CI, 1.2–1.9). The authors concluded that in the absence of trials and confounding factors notwithstanding, these observational data support improving glycemic control in younger patients prior to and during dialysis.

5.5   Management of Comorbidities

5.5.1   Diabetic Kidney Disease and Cardiovascular Complications

CVD (acute myocardial infarction, heart failure, cerebrovascular accidents, malignant arrhythmias, and sudden death) is the leading cause of death in the patients with overt DKD. Patients with diabetes on HD have the highest risk of cardiac death and nonfatal myocardial infarction. This risk is greater than in nondiabetic patients on HD (odds ratio [OR] 1.88) and in diabetic patients not on HD (OR 4.27) [39]. Silent myocardial ischemia (24 %) and left ventricular dilatation (49 %), as detected on myocardial perfusion imaging, are common among patients with diabetes initiating HD [40]. Additionally, diabetes is an independent risk factor for stroke in the HD population (OR 2.29) [41]. This increased risk profile is complicated by the often 'atypical' clinical presentation of myocardial ischemia in patients with diabetes undergoing dialysis due to the presence of autonomic neuropathy. In addition, vasomotor responses to change in volume status during dialysis are attenuated in diabetes, leading to more frequent symptomatic episodes of intradialytic hypotension and higher blood pressure both before and after a dialysis session [42].

5.5.2   Antidiabetic Therapy, Renal Impairment, and Heart Failure

The risk of heart failure (HF) is significantly increased in patients with diabetes and is particularly high in patients with diabetes and impaired renal function. In the SAVOR-TIMI 53 study, the risk of hospitalization for HF was increased by only 2.2 % in patients with an eGFR >50 mL/min/1.73 m^2, but 7.4 % in patients with moderate renal impairment (eGFR 30–50 mL/min/1.73 m^2) and 13 % in those with an eGFR <30 mL/min/1.73 m^2 [43]. Thus, in patients with advanced renal impairment, the effect of the various antihyperglycemic agents on HF must be assessed and balanced with their benefit in glucose reduction.

Metformin is now considered the safest therapeutic alternative for individuals with HF. Thiazolidinediones may cause HF, the main mechanism being fluid retention, and are generally contraindicated in patients with NYHA class III-IV HF [44]. Remarkably, when patients with CKD were analyzed in the pioglitazone CV outcome study (PROactive), those treated with pioglitazone were less likely to reach the combined endpoint of death, nonfatal MI, and nonfatal stroke versus placebo (HR 0.66; 95 % CI, 0.45–0.98) [45]. Thus, in patients with diabetes and a history of CVD, those with moderate renal impairment may benefit from pioglitazone (excluding patients with HF).

While insulin has been associated with an increased risk of HF in several studies, in the Outcome Reduction with an Initial Glargine INtervention (ORIGIN) trial, no such signal was observed [46]. The effect of DPP-4 inhibitors on the risk for hospitalization for HF has been extensively discussed in several observational studies and meta-analyses. The three randomized controlled trials of cardiovascular outcomes with saxagliptin, alogliptin, and sitagliptin vs. placebo (SAVOR, EXAMINE, TECOS) revealed contradictory results regarding the use of DPP-4 inhibitors and HF [43, 47, 48]. A significantly increased risk for HF was observed for saxagliptin, but not for alogliptin and sitagliptin. The discrepancy is unclear but might be explained by the fact that a considerable number of patients included in SAVOR were classified as CKD stages 3 and 4, whereas in TECOS, very few patients had CKD. Thus, DPP-4 inhibitors should only be carefully used in patients with diabetes and impaired renal function.

While the EMPA-REG Outcome study demonstrated a 35 % relative risk reduction of hospitalization for HF with the drug vs. placebo, it stands to be seen whether this is an SGLT2 drug class effect [27].

5.5.3   Antihypertensive Therapy

Based on the most recent Joint National Committee (JNC) 8 and KDIGO guidelines, BP levels in diabetes are recommended to be below 140/90 mmHg in order to reduce CVD mortality and slow CKD progression [49, 50]. The support for these BP levels is derived from a limited number of randomized trials among patients with diabetes with a focus on CVD event outcomes. However, there are no randomized controlled trials on BP levels that examine CKD events or focus on the failure of nocturnal dipping as confounders for the relationships between BP levels and CKD progression.

Lifestyle adjustments for elevated blood pressure consist of weight loss, if overweight or obese; a Dietary Approaches to Stop Hypertension (DASH)-style dietary pattern including reducing sodium and increasing potassium intake; moderation of alcohol intake; and increased physical activity. Pharmacological therapy for patients with diabetes and hypertension should comprise a regimen that includes either an ACE inhibitor or an ARB, but not both. If one class is not tolerated, the other should be substituted. Multiple-drug therapy (including a thiazide diuretic and ACE inhibitor/ ARB at maximal doses) is generally required to achieve blood pressure targets. If ACE inhibitors, ARBs, or diuretics are used, serum creatinine/eGFR and serum potassium levels have be monitored.

A network meta-analysis analyzed 63 randomized clinical trials of antihypertensive therapy in patients with diabetes with a follow-up of at least 12 months, reporting all-cause mortality, requirement for dialysis, or doubling of serum creatinine levels [51]. Of the 36,917 patients included in the study, 2400 deaths occurred, 766 patients required dialysis, and serum creatinine level doubled in 1099 patients. When compared with placebo, only ACE inhibitors significantly reduced the doubling of serum creatinine levels (OR 0.58; 95 % CI, 0.32–0.90), and only β-blockers showed a significant difference in mortality (OR 7.13; 95 % CI, 1.37–41.39) [51]. There was no statistical significance in the outcome of dialysis between the treatments. Although the beneficial effects of ACE inhibitors when compared with ARBs did not reach statistical significance, ACE inhibitors consistently showed higher probabilities of being in the superior-ranking positions among all three outcomes. While the protective effect of an ACE inhibitor plus a calcium channel blocker (CCB) compared with placebo was not statistically significant, the treatment ranking identified this combination therapy to have the greatest probability (73.9 %) for being the best treatment on reducing mortality, followed by ACE inhibitor plus diuretics (12.5 %), ACE inhibitors (2.0 %), CCBs (1.2 %), and ARBs (0.4 %) [51]. This meta-analysis confirmed the renoprotective effect and superiority of using ACE inhibitors in patients with diabetes, and available evidence is not able to show a better effect for ARBs. Considering the cost of drugs, the findings support the use of ACE inhibitors as the first-line antihypertensive agent in patients with diabetes. CCBs might be the preferred treatment in combination with ACE inhibitors if adequate BP control cannot be achieved by ACE inhibitors alone.

In a recent meta-analysis, the efficacy and safety of blood pressure-lowering agents in adults with diabetes and kidney disease was analyzed [52]. In total, 157 studies comprising 43,256 participants, mostly with type 2 diabetes and CKD, were included in the network meta-analysis. No drug regimen was found to be more effective than placebo for reducing all-cause mortality. However, when compared with placebo, ESRD was significantly less likely after dual treatment with an ARB and an ACE inhibitor (OR 0.62; 95 % CI, 0.43–0.90) and after ARB monotherapy (OR 0.77; 95 % CI, 0.65–0.92). No regimen significantly increased hyperkalemia or acute kidney injury, although combined ACE inhibitor and ARB treatment had the lowest rank among all interventions because of borderline increases in estimated risks of these harms (OR 2.69; 95 % CI, 0.97–7.47 for hyperkalemia; OR 2.69; 95 % CI, 0.98–7.38 for acute kidney injury) [52]. In conclusion, no blood pressure-lowering strategy prolonged survival in adults with diabetes and kidney disease. ACE inhibitors and ARBs, alone or in combination, were the most effective strategies against ESRD. Any benefits of combined ACE inhibitor and ARB treatment need to be balanced against potential harms of hyperkalemia and acute kidney injury.

5.5.4 Lipid-Lowering Strategies

DKD is accompanied by abnormalities in lipid metabolism related to decline in kidney function. The association between higher low-density lipoprotein cholesterol (LDL-C) and risk of myocardial infarction is weaker for people with lower baseline eGFR, despite higher absolute risk of myocardial infarction [53]. Thus, increased LDL-C seems to be less useful as a marker of coronary risk among people with CKD than in the general population. Clinical trials in nondialysis-dependent CKD suggest that CVD events and mortality are reduced with statins and statins + ezetimibe compared with placebo [54], whereby the beneficial effects do not seem to be modified by the presence or absence of diabetes. According to the recently released KDIGO guidelines, statins are recommended for all patients with diabetes and nondialysis-dependent CKD [55]. While the CVD benefits of statins are well established, statins do not alter kidney disease progression in those with preexisting CKD [56].

Although in earlier stages of CKD or in renal transplant recipients cholesterol lowering with statins appears to be effective, two prospective, randomized, placebo-controlled trials in patients undergoing HD did not show a significant benefit [57, 58]. In the AURORA study, the administration of rosuvastatin (10 mg/day) during a median follow-up of 3.8 years did not reduce the primary endpoint of combined cardiovascular events [57].

Similarly, in the 4D study, despite effective lowering of LDL-C (38 mg/dL, 42 %), atorvastatin did not improve the incidence rate of the primary endpoint in 1255 hemodialysis patients with type 2 diabetes [58]. Remarkably, a post hoc analysis of the 4D study showed that atorvastatin significantly reduced the rates of adverse outcomes in the highest quartile of LDL-C (>145 mg/dL) [59]. The HRs and 95 % CI were 0.69 (0.48–1.00) for the composite primary endpoint, 0.58 (0.34–0.99) for cardiac death, 0.48 (0.25–0.94) for sudden cardiac death, 0.62 (0.33– 1.17) for nonfatal myocardial infarction, 0.68 (0.47–0.98) for all cardiac events combined, and 0.72 (0.52–0.99) for death from all causes, respectively [59]. No such decrease was seen in any of the other quartiles of LDL-C at baseline. These findings suggest that statin treatment might be considered in patients with diabetes on HD with appropriately elevated LDL-C levels.

In the Study of Heart And Renal Protection (SHARP) trial, the efficacy of reducing LDL-C with simvastatin + ezetimibe (a selective cholesterol-absorption inhibitor) was analyzed in more than 9000 patients (23 % had diabetes and 33 % received dialysis) presenting with all stages of CKD [60]. A significant reduction of first major atherosclerotic events (i.e., nonfatal myocardial infarction or coronary death, nonhemorrhagic stroke, or arterial revascularization) was noted in patients allocated to simvastatin + ezetimibe, compared with placebo (RR 0.83, 95 % CI, 0.74–0.94; $P=0.002$). Risk reduction was very similar in patients with diabetes (0.78; 0.64–0.94) and without diabetes (0.86; 0.74–0.99). The risk reduction was significant in patients with CKD stages 3 and 4, but not in those with CKD stage 5 and in those requiring HD.

5.6   Management of Progressive Kidney Disease

In cases where avoidance of development of DKD has failed, the second approach is slowing disease progression. The most important therapeutic issues at this stage are control of hypertension and hyperglycemia.

Regarding hypertension, it was shown in large studies that approximately two-thirds of patients need antihypertensive combination therapy, with an average of three different classes needed to achieve BP goals [61–63]. The same is true in patients with DKD, and frequently more than three drugs are needed. As stated in many national and international guidelines, ACE inhibitors or ARBs may have unique advantages for initial and early treatment of hypertension [64, 65].

Another drug class shown to have antiproteinuric properties are the CCBs. Therefore, a CCB should be considered a meaningful antihypertensive combination partner in patients with DKD. For example, manidipine was shown to produce a BP reduction comparable to hydrochlorothiazide when added to candesartan, but the CCB was significantly superior with respect to reduction in urinary albumin excretion rate [66].

An additional aspect in the choice of antihypertensive combination therapy is to consider the patient's comorbidities. Antihypertensive drugs that are beneficial in certain comorbidities may be preferable in an individual patient (e.g., alpha-blockers in patients with hyperplasia of the prostate or β-blockers in patients with HF). A new issue that seems to be of importance placed on giving at least one antihypertensive at bedtime [64, 67]. Although currently none of the studies on bedtime antihypertensive therapy had progression of DKD as the primary endpoint, a positive outcome may be presumed from the published data. With regard to glucose control, all principles of treatment, as well as the treatment goals mentioned above, are applicable with respect to slowing disease progression.

Experimental drugs such as bardoxolone (a triterpenoid) target completely new inflammatory pathways and oxidative stress, which are thought to contribute to the development and progression of DKD, but failed in a large clinical trial because of a higher rate of CV events compared to placebo [68]. It is expected that future studies on the transcription factor Keap1-Nrf2 pathway will result in new therapeutic offers that delay, or even eventually improve, DKD [69].

5.6.1   Progression of Diabetic Kidney Disease from Stages 3 to 5

The timing and importance of follow-up visits for patients with CKD stage 3 depends on the individual patient's condition. A general approach recommended by the ADA is outlined in Table 5.1 [3]. A simple reminder is the "60/30 rule." Patients should be referred to a nephrologist if they have an eGFR of <60 mL/min to rule out important differential diagnoses other than DKD that may benefit from specific treatment. Patients must be referred to a physician experienced in kidney disease at an eGFR <30 mL/min to decide on the modality of RRT they are striving for, to prepare the respective access (fistula for HD or catheter placement for peritoneal dialysis), and/or to evaluate whether a patient is suitable for transplantation.

At follow-up visits, taking a recent patient history is advisable, including 'unrelated' nondiabetes-related problems such as infections, trauma, any undiagnosed issues, and medical treatments that have changed since the last visit (previous 3–6 months). Any new drugs and dosages (prescribed by other medical doctors) should be checked with respect to potential nephrotoxicity and dose adaption in relation to the present eGFR. Questions posed to patients should address loss of appetite, nausea, vomiting, changes in stool, shortness of breath, cardiac complaints (e.g., chest pain), and signs of neuropathy (e.g. pain, restless legs).

Routine clinical examination should include auscultation of the heart and lungs, inspection of the skin, search for edema (eyelids, legs, lung), and BP measurement.

TABLE 5.1 Management of chronic kidney disease in diabetes

GFR (mL/min/1.73 m^2)	Recommended management
All patients	Yearly measurement of Cr, UACR, and potassium

45–60	Referral to a nephrologist if possibility for nondiabetic kidney disease exists:
	    Duration of type 1 diabetes <10 years
	    Persistent albuminuria
	    Abnormal findings on renal ultrasound
	    Resistant hypertension
	    Rapid fall in eGFR
	    Active urinary sediment on urine microscopic examination

	Consider the need for dose adjustment of medications
	Monitor eGFR every 6 months
	Monitor electrolytes, bicarbonate, hemoglobin, calcium, phosphorus, and parathyroid hormone at least yearly
	Assure vitamin D sufficiency
	Consider bone density testing
	Referral for dietary counseling
30–44	Monitor eGFR every 3 months
	Monitor electrolytes, bicarbonate, hemoglobin, calcium, phosphorus, and parathyroid hormone, albumin and weight every 3–6 months
	Consider the need for dose adjustment of medications
<30	Referral to a nephrologist

Reproduced with permission from American Diabetes Association [3] ©American Diabetes Association

Cr creatinine, *eGFR* estimated glomerular filtration rate, *UACR* urine albumin to creatinine ratio

Measurement of body weight is advisable to recognize any weight gain due to fluid retention or weight loss due to uremia-related muscle wasting.

The potentially nephrotoxic effect of commonly used drugs, including over the counter medications (e.g. nonsteroidal anti-inflammatory drugs), should be discussed with the patient before they begin taking them. In addition, the importance of compliance and adherence to prescribed drugs should be discussed with the patient and his/her family repeatedly.

Laboratory tests for stage-3 patients should routinely include blood urea nitrogen (or blood urea), creatinine, eGFR, sodium, potassium, calcium, chloride, phosphate, bicarbonate, hemoglobin, and urinary albumin/creatinine ratio (UACR). Additional laboratory tests may be necessary with regard to special problems related to progressive renal insufficiency (Table 5.2).

While intervals in follow-up visits of 3–6 months may be appropriate in patients with stage 3a, at least monthly visits are required for patients with stage 5 diabetes-related CKD. In addition, patients with treatment noncompliance may benefit from more frequent visits and treatment discussions.

With disease progression, electrolyte disturbances such as hyperkalemia are expected. Hyperkalemia management includes dietary advice (reduce or avoid intake of fresh fruit, vegetables, juices, and salad in large amounts) and an investigation into potential metabolic acidosis, as hyperkalemia may result from an intracellular to extracellular shift of potassium only. Metabolic acidosis frequently occurs with advanced CKD and should be corrected where possible. Further, drugs that may cause hyperkalemia (renin–angiotensin inhibitors, potassium-sparing diuretics) have to be monitored and adapted, where appropriate.

Calcium-phosphate disturbances may also occur with advanced CKD, causing elevated phosphate and, subsequently, reduced calcium levels. In these patients, reduction or avoidance of food high in phosphate content is necessary. A practical approach is to reduce intake of meat and fish to no more than three times a week, as the instructions given in "grams of protein per day" may be difficult to follow. Prescribing phosphate binders may be necessary to pertain

TABLE 5.2 Recommended laboratory tests necessary for patients with advanced chronic kidney disease (CKD)

State	Laboratory tests
Renal anemia and other causes of anemia occurring in DKD-related CKD	Erythrocyte count, hemoglobin, mean cell hemoglobin (MCH), mean cell volume (MCV), when appropriate leucocyte count, thrombocyte count Iron, ferritin, transferrin, transferrin saturation, reticulocyte count, and/or percentage of hypochromic red cells Vitamin B12/folate level
Metabolic acidosis	pH, pO_2, pCO_2, actual bicarbonate
CKD–MBD (chronic kidney disease–mineral bone disorder)	Calcium, phosphate, parathyroid hormone
Vitamin D	Calcium, phosphate, vitamin D level
Nutritional status	Serum albumin (protein excretion rate, urinary albumin/creatinine ratio)

adequate food intake and control phosphate levels. Low calcium levels may be a reaction to high phosphate levels to maintain calcium x phosphate product in serum, but also may be the expression of a true calcium deficiency due to vitamin D deficiency. Thus, vitamin D levels should be determined. In case of deficiency, active vitamin D metabolites such as cholecalciferol (vitamin D_3) should be administered. Examples of the various drugs used for treating specific CKD-related conditions are given in Table 5.3.

5.7   Renal Replacement Therapy

5.7.1   Initiation

RRT is used to replace the kidneys' blood-filtering function and includes HD (e.g., hemofiltration, hemodiafiltration), peritoneal dialysis, and transplantation. Before initiation of RRT, both the disease and treatment burdens have to be considered and weighed against each other. Therefore, the decision to start this lifelong therapy is often a difficult one to make for physicians and patients. The decision has to be made in close collaboration of the patient, family members, and the nephrologist, as well as other medical doctors involved in the patient's care, such as a general practitioner. Consequently, RRT should be started when the risk and associated adverse effects on the patient's quality of life are clearly outweighed by the relief of uremic symptoms.

In line with guidelines, the medical decision to start RRT primarily depends on the presence (or absence) of uremia-related signs and symptoms and the patient's eGFR and its slope of decline over a recent period [70, 71]. In a remarkable study by Cooper and colleagues, it was shown that initiating dialysis at an eGFR of 10–15 mL/min/1.73 m^2 in comparison to an eGFR of 5–7 mL/min/1.73 m^2 did not improve survival or clinical outcomes [72]. In this trial, 34 % of the patients included had DKD-related ESRD. In case of ESRD-related symptoms, other causes should be ruled out and be treated medically. Only when symptoms are refractory to conservative treatment should RRT be started. However, eGFR calculated to the Modification of Diet in Renal Disease (MDRD) formula does not represent true GFR, as the formula is validated between 20 and 60 mL/min/1.73 m^2 only. Thus, a 24-h urine collection may be necessary with determination of the creatinine clearance. A clear-cut indication to start RRT urgently is the presence of uremic pericarditis or pleuritis, uremic encephalopathy, or severely symptomatic hyperkalemia.

Patients with DKD-related ESRD may differ somewhat in that severe volume overload refractory to high-dose diuretic therapy (not uremic symptoms) may prompt one to initiate RRT. Another issue is that other medical conditions unrelated to ESRD may alter the compensation mechanisms working in patients with advanced CKD. For instance, a flu-like infection or progressively decompensated HF may worsen a patient's overall condition markedly, and initiation of RRT may become necessary to compensate.

TABLE 5.3 Medical treatment of chronic kidney disease (CKD)-related problems

State	Examples of drugs potentially used for treatment[a] Generic name
Renal anemia	Erythropoiesis stimulating agents: Epoetin alfa Darbepoetin alfa
Iron deficiency	Oral: Ferrous sulfate Ferrous gluconate Iron polysaccharide Ferrous fumarate Intravenous: Sodium ferric gluconate complex in sucrose Ferric carboxymaltose Ferumoxytol
Vitamin B12 deficiency	Cyanocobalamin B12 Cyanocobalamin oral Cyanocobalamin intramuscular
Folic acid deficiency	Folic acid I-methylfolate Folic acid intravenous
Metabolic acidosis	Sodium bicarbonate Sodium citrate Citric acid Tromethamine
CKD–MBD (chronic kidney disease–mineral bone disorder)	
1. Phosphate binders	Calcium carbonate Calcium acetate Sevelamer hydrochloride Sevelamer carbonate Lanthanum carbonate Ferric citrate Sucroferric oxyhydroxide Aluminum hydroxide

(continued)

TABLE 5.3 (continued)

| State | Examples of drugs potentially used for treatment[a] |
	Generic name
2. Calcimimetic	Cinacalcet
3. Vitamin D	Vitamin D analogs
Vitamin D deficiency	Calcitriol oral
	Calcitriol intravenous
	Paricalcitol oral
	Doxercalciferol (D2)
	Ergocalciferol (D2)
	Cholecalciferol (D3)

[a]The examples given do not claim to be complete with regard to approval by regulatory authorities in the respective indication, nor do they indicate certain preferences in the treatment of a certain condition

Finally, patients with DKD-related ESRD and severe and/or multiple comorbid conditions with poor prognosis eventually may not be able to give informed consent due to cognitive impairment and/or high age; conservative treatment by a nephrologist without RRT may be considered a treatment option. However, this is related to reduced survival [73].

5.7.2   Hemodialysis Versus Peritoneal Dialysis

There are no randomized controlled studies comparing HD and peritoneal dialysis and its outcome in diabetic or nondiabetic patients. Therefore, the modality may be chosen according to the patient's preference. Consultation with a nephrologist is advisable early in the course of disease to rule out contraindications to either modality.

In general, comorbid conditions with a focus on ability to tolerate volume shifts may play a role. Patients with diabetes and autonomic neuropathy are more likely to develop hypotension during HD and, therefore, may benefit from the more gradual fluid removal seen with peritoneal dialysis. The presence of severe peripheral vascular disease with inability to place vascular access may favor peritoneal dialysis. However, an inappropriate home situation as well as visual impairment or reduced manual skillfulness may make peritoneal dialysis impossible to perform.

5.7.3   Living with Dialysis

Overall, the prognosis of patients with DKD-related ESRD has improved over the past two decades. Analyzing data from the Austrian Dialysis and Transplant Registry revealed an adjusted RR reduction in mortality of 33 % (HR 0.67; CI 95 %, 0.57–0.78; $P < 0.001$) in the cohort of patients with DKD starting dialysis in 2007–2008, when compared to the cohort initiating dialysis in 1997–1998 [11]. Nevertheless, survival is still markedly lower than in nondiabetic patients with ESRD.

As CVD accounts for more than half of deaths of patients undergoing dialysis, awareness has to be directed to even slight symptoms of angina, HF, and peripheral circulatory problems. Adequate diagnostic procedures should be initiated in a timely manner, followed by an appropriate therapy. With regard to coronary artery disease, a comparison of percutaneous intervention and coronary artery bypass grafting (CABG) was in favor of the latter procedure in multi-vessel disease [74]. The hazard ratio for CABG was 0.88 (95 % CI, 0.86–0.91) for the composite endpoint of death or myocardial infarction.

Routine dialysis visit should include a foot examination approximately every 3 months, or whenever appropriate. As neuropathy causes painless skin lesions and/or foot ulcers and vision may be impaired, this is an important responsibility for the healthcare professionals administering dialysis.

Kidney- or dialysis-related disturbances such as renal anemia, hyperkalemia and other electrolyte deviations, hyperphosphatemia with hyperparathyroidism, and vitamin D deficiency have to be managed adequately. The principles of treatment are identical to nondiabetic dialysis patients.

5.7.4   Transplantation

Kidney- or combined kidney–pancreas transplantation is a treatment option in patients with DKD that are suitable for transplantation. In general, a potential transplant recipient has to be free of malignant disease, active CVD, and infection. Individual transplant centers may have other specific requirements that need to be fulfilled by a potential candidate.

The choice of dialysis or kidney transplantation depends on many factors, including timely recognition of continued decline in renal function, resource availability, and patient comorbidity. In many countries, the overwhelming majority of patients with diabetes-related ESRD will initially be given RRT in the form of HD. Patients with diabetes and CKD experience a high incidence of CVD events and death, which increases after the initiation of dialysis therapy [75].

Thus, as survival and quality of life are superior with transplantation compared to dialysis, transplantation is worth striving for. An analysis of the USRDS data revealed an RR of 0.27 (95 % CI, 0.24–0.30) 18 months after transplantation in patients with diabetes in comparison to patients on dialysis on a transplant waiting list [76]. The gain in projected years of life with transplantation amounted to 11 years in patients with DKD in comparison to patients without transplantation.

The current recommendation for patients with type 1 diabetes is to undergo a simultaneous pancreas and kidney (SPK) transplant, while patients with type 2 diabetes typically receive a single kidney transplant (preferably a living donor kidney [LDK]). The optimal timing for transplantation for both patient populations is prior to needing dialysis (or with as little time spent on dialysis as possible) [77, 78].

Since the first reported successful pancreas transplant was performed in 1966, more than 35,000 pancreas transplantations have been reported to the International Pancreas Transplant Registry (IPTR), with more than 24,000 reported from centers in the United States [79, 80]. Pancreas transplantation is typically reserved for medically and surgically suitable candidates with type 1 diabetes with ESRD, where either SPK or pancreas-after-kidney transplantation (PAK) is performed.

It is well known that mortality due to CVD, particularly coronary artery disease (CAD), is high in patients with type 1 diabetes and ESRD. Very recently, authors from Norway analyzed whether normoglycemia achieved by successful SPK transplantation could improve long-term outcomes, compared with LDK transplantation [81]. In total, 486 patients with type 1 diabetes and ESRD who underwent an SPK ($n = 256$) or LDK ($n = 230$) transplant between 1983 and 2012 were followed for a median of 7.9 years. The adjusted HR for CVD-related deaths in SPK recipients compared with LDK recipients was 0.63 (95 % CI, 0.40–0.99; $P = 0.047$), while the reductions of all-cause and CAD-related mortality were not significant [82]. As expected when compared with the LDK group, SPK recipients were younger and received grafts from younger donors. CV mortality was higher in patients transplanted between 1983 and 1999, compared with those who received their grafts in subsequent years. The authors concluded that in patients with type 1 diabetes and ESRD, SPK transplantation was associated with reduced long-term CV mortality compared with LDK transplantation [81].

During the last 20 years, there has been an impressive improvement in laboratory testing procedures, surgical techniques, immunosuppressive therapy, surveillance, and treatment of recipients receiving a kidney transplant. In particular, cardiac assessment and primary and secondary prevention of CAD might have contributed to these improved outcomes. For SPK transplantation, the surgical technique has improved substantially with time, but surgical complications still cause a considerable rate of pancreas graft loss during the first weeks posttransplant; pancreas graft are inversely associated with patient survival. For kidney transplantation alone (KTA), graft loss due to early surgical complications is a very rare event. However, in

KTA transplantation, higher recipient and living donor age have been accepted in recent years and might have had a negative effect on survival.

Thus, when discussing transplantation with a patient, the potential complications related to transplantation (mainly surgery and immunosuppression) should be clearly considered and communicated. First, a slightly higher early mortality rate after transplantation is seen when compared to patients remaining on the transplantation waiting list [76]. Surgical complications such as bacterial, fungal, and viral infection, wound problems, and vascular thrombosis may also result in greater morbidity. More frequent hospitalizations may take place, especially during the first year after transplantation. With KTA, metabolic disturbances with hyperglycemia are seen and result from steroid- and calcineurin-related immunosuppression. Graft loss may occur, requiring a return to RRT. CVD is common after kidney transplantation and is much higher than in the general population [82]. Immunosuppressive agents (e.g., prednisolone, cyclosporine, and tacrolimus) have several detrimental effects on CV risk, including increased risk of hypertension, hyperlipidemia, and posttransplant diabetes mellitus.

In the United States, over the past 9 years, the number of pancreas transplantations has steadily declined from about 1500 in 2003 to 1000 in 2012 [83]. The fact that the number of pancreas transplants has declined by almost one-third is rather surprising because patient and graft survival rates during this time have increased. At 2 years, graft survival for SPK increased from 82 to 85 %; for PAK from 69 to 81 %; and for pancreas transplant alone (PTA), from 69 to 70 %. Significant decreases of graft losses owing technical and immunologic reasons for PAK and SPK accounted for the improvements in outcome. The declining number of pancreas transplants may be explained by several factors. During the last decade, significant improvements in the treatment of diabetes, in particular of patients with type 1 diabetes, have been seen in many countries. Diabetes education, self-monitoring of blood glucose, disease management programs, tight HbA1c monitoring, and modern devices including insulin pens and insulin pumps have significantly improved the prognosis of type 1 and type 2 diabetes [84, 85].

Many transplantation centers are reluctant to perform an SPK in patients older than 50 years of age and, according to the International Pancreas Transplant Registry, only 2 % of pancreas transplants are performed in patients older than 60 years of age [86].

Due to the decline of SPK procedures in patients with type 1 diabetes, some centers, particularly in the United States, are now also offering SPK to patients with type 2 diabetes. Margreiter et al. studied 216 patients undergoing SPK and found that patients with type 1 diabetes differed significantly from patients with type 2: three-quarters of patients with type 1 diabetes did not have findings of vascular disease, while three-quarters of patients with type 2 did [87]. The most common cause of pancreatic graft loss was rejection in patients with type 1 diabetes (vs. patient death in type 2). Importantly, patient and pancreas graft survival rates were not different at 5 years between the two groups [87]. Although the authors observed lower patient survival (90 vs. 96 %) in SPK patients with type 2 when compared to SPK patients with type 1 diabetes, overall patient survival of SPK patients with type 2 was still superior to patients undergoing KTA. Light et al. analyzed the long-term outcomes of 135 patients after SPK, of which 28 % had type 2 diabetes [88]. When the data were stratified by diabetes type, there was no observed difference in patient or pancreatic graft survival and long-term after 20 years [89], suggesting a similar patient and graft survival rate, regardless of diabetes type. In a recent review, Redfield et al. concluded that there is clearly a group of patients with type 2 diabetes who benefit from SPK, and both short-term and long-term outcomes are commensurate with patients with type 1 [90]. In conclusion, the benefits and disadvantages of transplantation have to be discussed extensively with the patient and always remain an individual decision apart from study and registry data.

References

1. Retnakaran R, Cull CA, Thorne KI, Adler AI, Holman RR. Risk factors for renal dysfunction in type 2 diabetes: UK Prospective Diabetes Study 74. Diabetes. 2006;55:1832–9.
2. Mottl AK, Kwon KS, Mauer M, Mayer-Davies EJ, Hogan SL, Kshirsagar AV. Normoalbuminuric diabetic kidney disease in the U.S. population. J Diabetes Complications. 2013;27:123–7.
3. American Diabetes Association. Summary of revisions. In: standards of medical care in diabetes – 2016. Diabetes Care. 2016;39(Suppl1):S4–5.
4. Menke A, Casagrande S, Geiss L, Cowie C. Prevalence of and trends in diabetes among adults in the United States, 1988–2012. JAMA. 2015;314:1021–9.
5. Bailey RA, Wang Y, Zhu V, Rupnow FT. Chronic kidney disease in US adults with type 2 diabetes: an updated national estimate of prevalence based on Kidney Disease: Improving Global Outcomes (KDIGO) staging. BMC Res Notes. 2014;7:415.
6. Kidney Disease: Improving Global Outcomes (KDIGO) CKD Work Group. KDIGO 2012 Clinical Practice Guideline for the Evaluation and Management of Chronic Kidney Disease. Kidney inter. 2013;3(Suppl.):1–150.
7. Noubiap JJ, Naidoo J, Kenge AP. Diabetic nephropathy in Africa: a systematic review. World J Diabetes. 2015;6:759–73.
8. United States Renal Data System 2014 Annual Data Report. Volume 1, Chapter 1: CKD in the general population. www.usrds.org/2014/view/Default.aspx. Accessed 7 Mar 2016.
9. United States Renal Data System 2014 Annual Data Report. Volume 2, Chapter 1: Incidence, prevalence, patient characteristics, and treatment modalities. www.usrds.org/2014/view/Default.aspx. Accessed 7 Mar 2016.
10. Nakai S, Hanafusa N, Masakane I, Taniguchi M, Hamano T, Shoji T, et al. An overview of regular dialysis treatment in Japan (as of 31 December 2012). Ther Apher Dial. 2014;18:535–602.
11. Prischl FC, Auinger M, Säemann M, Mayer G, Rosenkranz AR, Wallner M, Kramar R, Austrian Dialysis and Transplant Registry. Diabetes-related end stage renal disease in Austria 1965–2013. Nephrol Dial Transplant. 2015;30:1920–7.
12. Pippias M, Jager KJ, Kramer A, Leivestad T, Sánchez MB, Caskey FJ, et al. The changing trends and outcomes in renal replacement therapy: data from the ERA-EDTA Registry. Nephrol Dial Transplant. 2016;31(5):831–41.

13. Pippias M, Stel VS, Abad Diez JM, Afentakis N, Herrero-Calvo JA, Arias M, et al. Renal replacement therapy in Europe: a summary of the 2012 ERA-EDTA Registry annual report. Clin Kidney J. 2015;8:248–61.
14. European Renal Association (ERA)-European Dialysis and Transplant Association Registry (EDTA). ERA-EDTA Registry Annual Report 2012. Academic Medical Center, Department of Medical Informatics, Amsterdam, 2014. www.era-edta-reg.org/files/annualreports/pdf/AnnRep2012.pdf. Accessed 7 Mar 2016.
15. Gregg EW, Cheng YJ, Saydah S, Cowie C, Garfield S, Geiss L, et al. Trends in death rates among US adults with and without diabetes between 1997 and 2006. Diabetes Care. 2012;35:1252–7.
16. deBoer IH, Rue TC, Hall YN, Heagerty PJ, Weiss NS, Himmelfarb J, et al. Temporal trends in the prevalence of diabetic kidney disease in the United States. J Am Med Assoc. 2011;305:2532–9.
17. Biesenbach G, Janko O, Zazgornik J. Similar rate of progression in the predialysis phase in type 1 and type 2 diabetes mellitus. Nephrol Dial Transplant. 1994;9:1097–102.
18. Teng J, Dwyer KM, Hill P, See E, Ekinci EI, Jerums G, et al. Spectrum of renal disease in diabetes. Nephrology. 2014;19:528–36.
19. Schernthaner G, Ritz E, Schernthaner GH. Strict glycaemic control in diabetic patients with CKD or ESRD: beneficial or deadly? Nephrol Dial Transplant. 2010;25:2044–7.
20. Arnouts P, Bolignano D, Nistor I, Bilo H, Gnudi L, Heaf J, et al. Glucose-lowering drugs in patients with chronic kidney disease: a narrative review on pharmacokinetic properties. Nephrol Dial Transplant. 2014;29:1284–300.
21. Avogaro A, Schernthaner G. Achieving glycemic control in patients with type 2 diabetes and renal impairment. Acta Diabetol. 2013;50:283–91.
22. Groop PH, Del Prato S, Taskinen MR, Owens DR, Gong Y, Crowe S, et al. Linagliptin treatment in subjects with type 2 diabetes with and without mild-to-moderate renal impairment. Diabetes Obes Metab. 2014;16:560–8.
23. Schernthaner G, Barnett AH, Patel S, Hehnke U, von Eynatten M, Woerle HJ. Safety and efficacy of the dipeptidyl peptidase-4 inhibitor linagliptin in elderly patients with type 2 diabetes: a comprehensive analysis of data from 1331 individuals aged ≥ 65 years. Diabetes Obes Metab. 2014;16:1078–86.

24. Whalen K, Miller S, Onge ES. The role of sodium-glucose co-transporter 2 inhibitors in the treatment of type 2 diabetes. Clin Ther. 2015;37:1150–66.
25. Schernthaner G, Gross JL, Rosenstock J, Guarisco M, Fu M, Yee J, et al. Canagliflozin compared with sitagliptin for patients with type 2 diabetes who do not have adequate glycemic control with metformin plus sulfonylurea: a 52-week randomized trial. Diabetes Care. 2013;36:2508–15.
26. Gilbert RE. Sodium-glucose linked transporter-2 inhibitors: potential for renoprotection beyond blood glucose lowering? Kidney Int. 2014;86:693–700.
27. Zinman B, Wanner C, Lachin JM, Fitchett D, Bluhmki E, Hantel S, et al. Empagliflozin, cardiovascular outcomes, and mortality in type 2 diabetes. N Engl J Med. 2015;373:2117–28.
28. Wanner C, Lachin JM, Fitchett DH, Inzucchi SE, von Eynatten M, Mattheus M, et al. Empagliflozin and cardiovascular outcomes in patients with type 2 diabetes and chronic kidney disease. JASN. 2015;26(Suppl B1):1133.
29. Schernthaner G, Schernthaner-Reiter MH. Therapy: risk of metformin use in patients with T2DM and advanced CKD. Nat Rev Endocrinol. 2015;11:697–9.
30. Hung SC, Chang YK, Liu JS, Hsu CC, Tarng DC. Metformin use and mortality in patients with advanced chronic kidney disease: national, retrospective, observational, cohort study. Lancet Diabetes Endocrinol. 2015;3:605–14.
31. Roussel R, Lorraine J, Rodriguez A, Salaun-Martin C. Overview of data concerning the safe use of antihyperglycemic medications in type 2 diabetes mellitus and chronic kidney disease. Adv Ther. 2015;32:1029–64.
32. Morioka T, Emoto M, Tabata T, Shoji T, Tahara H, Kishimoto H, et al. Glycemic control is a predictor of survival for diabetic patients on hemodialysis. Diabetes Care. 2001;24:909–13.
33. Oomichi T, Emoto M, Tabata T, Morioka T, Tsujimoto Y, Tahara H, et al. Impact of glycemic control on survival of diabetic patients on chronic regular hemodialysis: a 7-year observational study. Diabetes Care. 2006;29:1496–500.
34. Hayashino Y, Fukuhara S, Akiba T, Akizawa T, Asano Y, Saito A, et al. Diabetes, glycaemic control and mortality risk in patients on haemodialysis: the Japan Dialysis Outcomes and Practice Pattern Study. Diabetologia. 2007;50:1170–7.

35. Kalantar-Zadeh K, Kopple JD, Regidor DL, Jing J, Shinaberger CS, Aronovitz J, et al. A1C and survival in maintenance hemodialysis patients. Diabetes Care. 2007;30:1049–55.
36. Drechsler C, Krane V, Ritz E, März W, Wanner C. Glycemic control and cardiovascular events in diabetic hemodialysis patients. Circulation. 2009;120:2421–8.
37. Hill CJ, Maxwell AP, Cardwell CR, Freeman BI, Tonelli M, Emoto M, et al. Glycated hemoglobin and risk of death in diabetic patients treated with hemodialysis: a meta-analysis. Am J Kidney Dis. 2014;63:84–94.
38. Adler A, Casula A, Steenkamp R, Fogarty D, Wilkie M, Tomlinson L, et al. Association between glycemia and mortality in diabetic individuals on renal replacement therapy in the U.K. Diabetes Care. 2014;37:1304–11.
39. Le Feuvre C, Borentain M, Beygui F, Helft G, Batisse JP, Metzger JP. Comparison of short- and long-term outcomes of coronary angioplasty in patients with and without diabetes mellitus and with and without hemodialysis. Am J Cardiol. 2003;92:721–5.
40. Momose M, Babazono T, Kondo C, Kobayashi H, Nakajima T, Kusakabe K. Prognostic significance of stress myocardial ECG-gated perfusion imaging in asymptomatic patients with diabetic chronic kidney disease on initiation of haemodialysis. Eur J Nucl Med Mol Imaging. 2009;36:1315–21.
41. Sánchez-Perales C, Vázquez E, García-Cortés MJ, Borrego J, Polaina M, Guitierrez CP, et al. Ischaemic stroke in incident dialysis patients. Nephrol Dial Transplant. 2010;25:3343–8.
42. Davenport A, Cox C, Thuraisingham R. Blood pressure control and symptomatic intradialytic hypotension in diabetic haemodialysis patients: a cross-sectional survey. Nephron Clin Pract. 2008;109:c65–71.
43. Udell JA, Bhatt DL, Braunwald E, Cavender MA, Mosenzon O, Steg PG, et al. Saxagliptin and cardiovascular outcomes in patients with type 2 diabetes and moderate or severe renal impairment: observations from the SAVOR-TIMI 53 Trial. Diabetes Care. 2015;38:696–705.
44. Erdmann E, Charbonnel B, Wilcox RG, Skene AM, Massi-Benedetti M, Yates J, et al. Pioglitazone use and heart failure in patients with type 2 diabetes and preexisting cardiovascular disease: data from the PROactive study (PROactive 08). Diabetes Care. 2007;30:2773–8.

45. Schneider CA, Ferrannini E, Defronzo R, Schernthaner G, Yates J, Erdmann E. Effect of pioglitazone on cardiovascular outcome in diabetes and chronic kidney disease. J Am Soc Nephrol. 2008;19:182–7.
46. ORIGIN Trial Investigators, Gerstein HC, Bosch J, Dagenais GR, Díaz R, Jung H, et al. Basal insulin and cardiovascular and other outcomes in dysglycemia. N Engl J Med. 2012;367:319–28.
47. Zannad F, Cannon CP, Cushman WC, Bakris GL, Menon V, Perez AT, et al. Heart failure and mortality outcomes in patients with type 2 diabetes taking alogliptin versus placebo in EXAMINE: a multicentre, randomised, double-blind trial. Lancet. 2015;385:2067–76.
48. Green JB, Bethel A, Armstrong PW, Buse JB, Engel SS, Garg J, et al. Effect of sitagliptin on cardiovascular outcomes in type 2 diabetes. N Engl J Med. 2015;373:232–42.
49. Kidney Disease International Global Outcomes (KDIGO). Clinical practice guideline for the management of blood pressure in chronic kidney disease. Kidney Int. 2012;Suppl 2:337–414.
50. James PA, Oparil S, Carter BL, Cushman WC, Dennison-Himmelfarb C, Handler J, et al. 2014 evidence-based guideline for the management of high blood pressure in adults: report from the panel members appointed to the Eighth Joint National Committee (JNC 8). JAMA. 2014;311:507–20.
51. Wu HY, Huang JW, Lin HJ, Liao WC, Peng YS, Hung KY, et al. Comparative effectiveness of renin-angiotensin system blockers and other antihypertensive drugs in patients with diabetes: systematic review and bayesian network meta-analysis. BMJ. 2013;347:f6008.
52. Palmer SC, Mavridis D, Navarese E, Craig JC, Tonelli M, Salanti G, et al. Comparative efficacy and safety of blood pressure-lowering agents in adults with diabetes and kidney disease: a network meta-analysis. Lancet. 2015;385:2047–56.
53. Tonelli M, Muntner P, Lloyd A, Manns B, Klarenbach S, Pannu N, et al. Association between LDL-C and risk of myocardial infarction in CKD. J Am Soc Nephrol. 2013;24:979–86.
54. Palmer SC, Craig JC, Navaneethan SD, Tonelli M, Pellegrini F, Strippoli GF. Benefits and harms of statin therapy for persons with chronic kidney disease: a systematic review and meta-analysis. Ann Intern Med. 2012;157:263–75.

55. Wanner C, Tonelli M, Kidney Disease: Improving Global Outcomes (KDIGO) Lipid Guideline Development Work Group Members. KDIGO Clinical Practice Guideline for Lipid Management in CKD: summary of recommendation statements and clinical approach to the patient. Kidney Int. 2014;85:1303–9.
56. Haynes R, Lewis D, Emberson J, Reith C, Agodoa L, Cass A, et al; SHARP Collaborative Group. Effects of lowering LDL cholesterol on progression of kidney disease. J Am Soc Nephrol. 2014;25:1825–33.
57. Fellström BC, Jardine AG, Schmieder RE, Holdaas H, Bannister K, Beutler J, AURORA Study Group. Rosuvastatin and cardiovascular events in patients undergoing hemodialysis. N Engl J Med. 2009;360:1395–407.
58. Wanner C, Krane V, März W, Olschewski M, Mann JF, Ruf G, et al. Atorvastatin in patients with type 2 diabetes mellitus undergoing hemodialysis. N Engl J Med. 2005;353:238–48.
59. März W, Genser B, Drechsler C, Krane V, Grammer TB, Ritz E, et al. Atorvastatin and low-density lipoprotein cholesterol in type 2 diabetes mellitus patients on hemodialysis. Clin J Am Soc Nephrol. 2011;6:1316–25.
60. Baigent C, Landray MJ, Reith C, Emberson J, Wheeler DC, Tomson C, et al. SHARP Investigators. The effects of lowering LDL cholesterol with simvastatin plus ezetimibe in patients with chronic kidney disease (Study of Heart and Renal Protection): a randomised placebo-controlled trial. Lancet. 2011;377:2181–92.
61. Bakris GL, Williams M, Dworkin L, Elliott WJ, Epstein M, Toto R, et al. Preserving renal function in adults with hypertension and diabetes: a consensus approach. National Kidney Foundation Hypertension and Diabetes Executive Committees Working Group. Am J Kidney Dis. 2000;36:646–61.
62. Lewis EJ, Hunsicker LG, Clarke WR, Berl T, Pohl MA, Lewis JB, et al. Collaborative Working Group. Renoprotective effect of the angiotensin-receptor antagonist irbesartan in patients with nephropathy due to type 2 diabetes. N Engl J Med. 2001;345:851–60.
63. Cushman WC, Ford CE, Cutler JA, Margolis KL, Davis BR, Grimm RH, et al., ALLHAT Collaborative Research Group. Success and predictors of blood pressure control in diverse North American settings: the antihypertensive and lipid-lowering treatment to prevent heart attack trial (ALLHAT). J Clin Hypertens. 2002;4:393–404.

64. American Diabetes Association. Cardiovascular disease and risk management. Sec.8. In: Standards of medical care in diabetes – 2016. Diabetes Care. 2016;39(Suppl. 1):S60–71.
65. Garber AJ, Abrahamson MJ, Barzilay JI, Blonde L, Bloomgarden ZT, Bush MA, et al. Consensus statement by the American Association of Clinical Endocrinologists and American College of Endocrinology on the comprehensive type 2 diabetes management algorithm – 2016 executive summary. Endocr Pract. 2016;22:84–113.
66. Fogari R, Corradi L, Zoppi A, Lazzari P, Mugellini A, Preti P, et al. Addition of manidipine improves the antiproteinuric effect of candesartan in hypertensive patients with type II diabetes and microalbuminuria. Am J Hypertension. 2007;20:1092–6.
67. Hermida R, Ayala DE, Mojon A, Fernandez JR. Influence of time of day of blood pressure lowering treatment on cardiovascular risk in hypertensive patients with type 2 diabetes. Diabetes Care. 2011;34:1270–6.
68. deZeeuw D, Akizawa T, Audhya P, Bakris GL, Chin M, Christ-Schmidt H, et al. Bardoxolone methyl in type 2 diabetes and stage 4 chronic kidney disease. N Engl J Med. 2013;369:2492–503.
69. Zoja C, Benigni A, Remuzzi G. The Nrf2 pathway in the progression of kidney disease. Nephrol Dial Transplant. 2014;29 Suppl 1:i19–24.
70. National Kidney Foundation. KDOQI clinical practice guidelines for hemodialysis adequacy: 2015 update. Am J Kidney Dis. 2015;66:884–930.
71. Tattersall J, Dekker F, Heimbürger O, Jager KJ, Lameire N, Lindley E, et al.; ERBP Advisory Board. When to start dialysis: updated guidance following publication of the Initiating Dialysis Early and Late (IDEAL) study. Nephrol Dial Transplant. 2011;26:2082–6.
72. Cooper BA, Branley P, Bulfone L, Collins JF, Craig JC, Fraenkel MB, et al; IDEAL Study. A randomized, controlled trial of early versus late initiation of dialysis. N Engl J Med. 2010;363:609–19.
73. Murtagh FE, Marsh JE, Donohoe P, Ekbal NJ, Sheerin NS, Harris FE. Dialysis or not? A comparative survival study of patients over 75 years with chronic kidney disease stage 5. Nephrol Dial Transplant. 2007;22:1955–62.
74. Chang TI, Shilane D, Kazi DS, Montez-Rath ME, Hlatky MA, Winkelmayer WC. Multivessel coronary artery bypass grafting versus percutaneous coronary intervention in ESRD. J Am Soc Nephrol. 2012;23:2042–9.

75. Foley RN, Murray AM, Li S, Herzog CA, McBean Am, Eggers PW, et al. Chronic kidney disease and the risk for cardiovascular disease, renal replacement, and death in the United States Medicare population, 1998 to 1999. J Am Soc Nephrol. 2005;16:489–95.
76. Wolfe RA, Ashby VB, Milford EL, Ojo AO, Ettenger RE, Agodoa LY, et al. Comparison of mortality in all patients on dialysis, patients on dialysis awaiting transplantation, and recipients of a first cadaveric transplant. N Engl J Med. 1999;341:1725–39.
77. Meier-Kriesche HU, Kaplan B. Waiting time on dialysis as the strongest modifiable risk factor for renal transplant outcomes: a paired donor kidney analysis. Transplantation. 2002;74:1377–81.
78. Son YK, Oh JS, Kim SM, Jm J, Shin YH, Kim JK. Clinical outcome of preemptive kidney transplantation in patients with diabetes mellitus. Transplant Proc. 2010;42:3497–502.
79. Kelly WD, Lillehei RC, Merkel FK, Idezuki Y, Goetz FC. Allotransplantation of the pancreas and duodenum along with the kidney in diabetic nephropathy. Surgery. 1967;61:827–37.
80. Gruessner AC. 2011 update on pancreas transplantation: comprehensive trend analysis of 25,000 cases followed up over the course of twenty-four years at the International Pancreas Transplant Registry (IPTR). Rev Diabet Stud. 2011;8:6–16.
81. Lindahl JP, Hartmann A, Aakhus S, Endresen K, Midtvedt K, Holdass H, et al. Long-term cardiovascular outcomes in type 1 diabetic patients after simultaneous pancreas and kidney transplantation compared with living donor kidney transplantation. Diabetologia. 2016;59(4):844–52.
82. Jardine AG, Gaston RS, Fellstrom BC, Holdaas H. Prevention of cardiovascular disease in adult recipients of kidney transplants. Lancet. 2011;378:1419–27.
83. Gruessner AC, Gruessner RW. Declining numbers of pancreas transplantations but significant improvements in outcome. Transplant Proc. 2014;46:1936–7.
84. Lind M, Svensson AM, Kosiborod M, Gudbjörnsdottir S, Pivodic A, Wedel H, et al. Glycemic control and excess mortality in type 1 diabetes. N Engl J Med. 2014;371:1972–82.
85. Tancredi M, Rosengren A, Svensson AM, Kosiborod M, Pivodic A, Gudbjörnsdottir S, et al. Excess mortality among persons with type 2 diabetes. N Engl J Med. 2015;373:1720–32.

86. Fourtounas C. Transplant options for patients with type 2 diabetes and chronic kidney disease. World J Transplant. 2014;4:102–10.

87. Margreiter C, Resch T, Oberhuber R, Aigner F, Maier H, Sucher R, et al. Combined pancreas-kidney transplantation for patients with end-stage nephropathy caused by type-2 diabetes mellitus. Transplantation. 2013;95:1030–6.

88. Light JA, Barhyte DY. Simultaneous pancreas-kidney transplants in type I and type II diabetic patients with end-stage renal disease: similar 10-year out-comes. Transplant Proc. 2005;37:1283–4.

89. Light J, Tucker M. Simultaneous pancreas kidney transplants in diabetic patients with end-stage renal disease: the 20-yr experience. Clin Transplant. 2013;27:E256–63.

90. Redfield RR, Scalea JR, Odorico JS. Simultaneous pancreas and kidney transplantation: current trends and future directions. Curr Opin Organ Transplant. 2015;20:94–102.

Chapter 6
Managing Diabetic Nephropathies in Clinical Practice: Emerging and Future Therapies

Colleen Majewski and George L. Bakris

6.1 Introduction

Diabetes mellitus is a serious chronic disease that will result in a diverse range of complications if not properly treated early in its course. This is especially true for people at risk of developing diabetic kidney disease (DKD), which is roughly about 30 % of patients with diabetes. In the past two decades, several new therapies have been approved to control glucose levels in diabetes mellitus. These advances have resulted in a slowing of nephropathy progression in some patients by 70 %, from an average of 5–6 mL/min/year to 2 mL/min/year [1]. This is because some of these treatments (e.g., sodium–glucose co-transporter 2 [SGLT2] inhibitors) have secondary benefits that affect the onset of nephropathy independent of effects on the renin–angiotensin system or hemodynamic changes. Given the unique action of SGLT2 inhibitors on the proximal tubule of the kidney, these agents are now also being examined for effects on slowing the progression of DKD. A dual SGLT1/SGLT2 inhibitor is also on the horizon. While not yet approved for general use, this subclass of medicine may provide even more effective glucose control and benefits on blood pressure. Apart from SGLT2 inhibitors, a more concentrated insulin glargine (U-300) has been approved for use in diabetes mellitus within the last year, with specific reference to people with kidney disease. Additionally, a new formulation of metformin appears to be safe to use in Stages 3 and 4 chronic kidney disease (CKD) because of its unique site of action localized to the small intestine. All of these agents and the data surrounding their development will be discussed in this chapter.

There are three major ongoing clinical outcome trials (SONAR, CREDENCE, and FIDELIO-DKD) focused on halting the progression of DKD [2–4]. These studies are actively recruiting and have end points focused on CKD progression and changes in estimated glomerular filtration rate (eGFR) and development of end-stage renal disease (ESRD). It should be noted the agents in these studies (i.e., atrasentan, pyridorin, and finerenone) do not appear to directly affect glycemic control and will need to be used in combination with antidiabetic treatments. These trials will also be discussed in this chapter.

6.2   Sodium–Glucose Co-transporter 2 Inhibitors

SGLT2 inhibitors are a relatively new class of agents used to control blood sugar in type 2 diabetes mellitus (T2DM). An SGLT2 transporter mediates glucose reabsorption in the proximal tubule and regulates 90 % of all glucose reabsorption by the kidney [5]. Thus, SGLT2 inhibitors act by competitive and selective inhibition of the SGLT2 transporter. Patients with T2DM overexpress SGLT2 receptors, a compensatory mechanism to promote glucose reabsorption, and the use of these medications in T2DM decreases the renal glucose threshold, leading to an increase in urinary glucose excretion. This glycosuric effect also may lead to some weight loss and a small reduction in blood pressure, due to the mild natriuretic and osmotic diuretic effects. These agents are approved to treat T2DM, but they are also being used off-label in patients with type 1 diabetes mellitus (T1DM) to try to reduce insulin requirements. SGLT2 inhibitors canagliflozin, dapagliflozin, and empagliflozin have been approved by the several SGLT2 inhibitors, have now been approved by the Food and Drug Administration (FDA) and other major advisory bodies, and are currently available in several countries. In addition to these, ipragliflozin and tofogliflozin are available in Japan.

Numerous trials on SGLT2 inhibitors have demonstrated significant reductions in glycated hemoglobin (HbA1c) levels in patients with T2DM [6]. Dapagliflozin and empagliflozin are highly selective for the SGLT2 transporters, whereas canagliflozin also has some inhibition of SGLT1 transporters located in the distal portion of the proximal tubule and the gut. SGLT1 transporters are responsible for approximately 10 % of renal glucose reabsorption and contribute to intestinal glucose absorption. Canagliflozin has been shown to delay intestinal glucose absorption, in addition to inhibiting renal glucose reabsorption [7]. While these medications have been used safely in patients with Stage 3 CKD (eGFR down to 30 mL/min), the glycemic reduction response to the SGLT2 inhibitors declines with decreasing kidney function, as a decrease in eGFR results in a decrease in urinary glucose excretion [6]. Canagliflozin has been approved for use in patients with eGFR >45 mL/min/1.73 m^2, with dose limited to 100 mg once daily in patients with eGFR 45–<60 mL/min/1.73 m^2. Empagliflozin can also be used in patients with an eGFR down to 45 mL/min/1.73 m^2, while dapagliflozin is approved in patients with an eGFR down ≥60 mL/min/1.73 m^2. Regular assessment of renal function is recommended with use of any of these SGLT2 inhibitors.

The upcoming CREDENCE trial will examine the effects of canagliflozin on slowing progression CKD in patients with diabetes and is currently enrolling patients [3]. The goal of this study is to assess whether canagliflozin has a renal and vascular protective effect, causing a reduction of the progression of renal impairment relative to placebo in participants with T2DM, Stage 2 or 3 CKD, and very high albuminuria (>300 mg/day), who are receiving standard of care, including a maximum tolerated labeled daily dose of an angiotensin-converting enzyme (ACE) inhibitor or angiotensin receptor blocker (ARB). Trial data is not expected until 2019. Another study of canagliflozin showed a clear benefit for lowering blood pressure in patients with eGFR $\geq$30 mL/min/1.73 m^2 but has not yet been approved for use in these patients [8].

Due to reduced glycemic control based on level of kidney function, further studies have attempted to determine the renal effects of SGLT2 inhibitors. Ojima et al. treated streptozocin-induced diabetic rats with empagliflozin for 4 weeks. In addition to improving blood glucose levels, the rats treated with empagliflozin had decreased levels of markers of oxidative stress in the diabetic kidney [9]. Specifically, levels of advanced glycation end products (AGE) and receptor advanced glycation end products (RAGE) were significantly lowered [9].

Hyperfiltration is considered an early marker of risk for diabetic nephropathy and is associated with abnormally high plasma glucose levels [10]. Cherney et al. investigated the effects of empagliflozin 25 mg daily on renal hyperfiltration in patients with T1DM [11]. 40 subjects completed the study, 13 with normofiltering kidneys, and 27 with renal hyperfiltration. The subjects were treated with empagliflozin for 8 weeks, and in the subjects with renal hyperfiltration, treatment with empagliflozin for 8 weeks resulted in a significant reduction in hyperfiltration during both clamped euglycemic and hyperglycemic conditions [11]. The changes in tubuloglomerular feedback examined by Cherney relate to the natriuretic effects of the SGLT2 agents and wane over time as a new level of glucose homeostasis is achieved [11].

Another factor important in assessing volume status in diabetes is atrial natriuretic peptide (ANP) [12]. Diabetes is a volume-expanded state for many reasons, and a compensatory increase in ANP is well documented. ANP results in suppression of the renin–angiotensin system and contributes to hyperfiltration. Animal studies have demonstrated that phlorizin, a nonspecific inhibitor of SGLT1 and SGLT2, via its osmotic diuretic and natriuretic effects, reduces ANP and reestablishes a new volume status in animals over 2–3 days [13]. This improvement in volume also contributes to reductions in blood pressure [14, 15]. Additionally, experimental animal models have demonstrated a restoration of tubuloglomerular feedback that is altered in renal hyperfiltration [16]. However, due to the poor tolerability of phlorizin in humans, the effects of this drug on renal hyperfiltration are not yet known, and more studies are needed.

Common side effects of SGLT2 inhibitors include genital mycotic infections and urinary tract infections. The more serious side effect of euglycemic diabetic ketoacidosis (DKA) has been reported in both patients with T1DM and T2DM [17]. The practitioner should have a high index of suspicion for euglycemic DKA, especially in patients who may be volume depleted and have reduced their insulin dosage. Additionally, if a patient reports headache, nausea, vomiting, or malaise on these agents, this may be a life-threatening condition that requires immediate treatment [17].

6.3   Novel Therapies in Development

6.3.1   Endothelin-A Receptor Antagonists

The Phase II RADAR trial successfully tested the hypothesis that low-dose atrasentan, a selective endothelin-A receptor antagonist, reduces albuminuria and slows nephropathy progression [18]. In it, a low dose of atrasentan (0.75 mg/day) was found to lower albuminuria by 36 % without major side effects in patients with T2DM with nephropathy who were treated with the maximal tolerated labeled dose of ACE inhibitors/ARBs. A higher dose of atrasentan (1.25 mg/day) had a similar albuminuria-lowering effect but produced more edema and weight gain [19].

Following on from these results, the Phase III SONAR trial is investigating atrasentan in patients with type 2 diabetes, hypertension, and diabetic nephropathy [2]. Subjects in this trial are also on a maximally tolerated ACE inhibitor or ARB dose prior to entering the study and have an eGFR of

25–75 mL/min/1.73 m^2 and a urine albumin/creatinine ratio (UACR) ≥300 mg/g. The primary outcome measures of the SONAR trial are the time to the first occurrence of a component of the composite renal endpoint: doubling of serum creatinine (SCr) (confirmed by a 30-day serum creatinine) or the onset of ESRD (defined in the study as an eGFR less >15 mL/min/1.73 m^2 [confirmed by a 90-day eGFR], patient receiving chronic dialysis, requiring renal transplantation, or renal death) [2]. Subjects are first entered into an enrichment period and treated with atrasentan, while a subset of subjects are enrolled in a double-blind component and randomized to atrasentan or placebo.

6.3.2   Inflammatory Response Inhibitors

Microvascular injury is the fundamental cause of DKD. Pyridorin (pyridoxamine dihydrochloride) is a novel small molecule with a chemical structure similar to, but distinct from, vitamin B6 (pyridoxine) that has an inhibitory effect on oxidative stress and reduces AGE formation, which are known to damage protein structure, reduce function, and lead to vascular injury. Additionally, pyridorin inhibits redox metal-binding activity that blocks oxidation of Amadori intermediates to AGEs.

PIONEER was a Phase III trial to explore the effects of pyridorin on the progression of diabetic nephropathy [20]. The primary outcome measures include time to composite end point of ≥50 % increase in serum creatinine (SCr) from baseline or ESRD (defined as the initiation of permanent dialysis, receiving a kidney transplant, or a SCr value ≥6.0 mg/dL [530 µmol/L] with a second SCr confirmation value ≥6.0 mg/dL [530 µmol/L] obtained 4–6 weeks later). The secondary outcome measures of this trial are time to the composite end point greater than or equal to a 100 % SCr increase or ESRD. However, due to funding constraints, the trial was prematurely terminated, not related to any adverse effects or other problems.

6.3.3   Mineralocorticoid Receptor Agonists

Two separate Phase III trials (FIDELIO-DKD and FIGARO-DKD) are now recruiting participants to examine the effects of finerenone, a steroidal antimineralocorticoid, on the progression of diabetic nephropathy, as well as cardiovascular outcomes [4, 21]. The primary outcome for FIDELIO-DKD (and secondary endpoint for FIGARO) is time to the first occurrence of the composite endpoint of onset of kidney failure, a sustained decrease of eGFR $\geq$40 % from baseline over at least 4 weeks, and renal death. Trial data for these studies are also expected in 2019.

6.4   Dual SGLT1/SGLT2 Inhibitor

Sotagliflozin, a dual SGLT1 and SGLT2 inhibitor, is another emerging therapy for treating patients with T2DM. SGLT1 is the major transporter for the absorption of glucose and galactose in the intestine [22]. SGLT1 knockout mice have demonstrated a dramatic reduction in postprandial glucose and an increase in glucagon-like peptide 1 (GLP-1) produced by L cells, which is involved in glucose control [23]. Inhibiting SGLT1 has also been shown to stimulate the release of polypeptide tyrosine tyrosine (PYY), which is involved in appetite control [24]. Adverse events in the knockout mice included watery or unformed stools when fed a diet of glucose or galactose. However, mice with a partial knockout of SGLT1 had normal stools when fed glucose and still maintained an increase in glucose load to the distal small intestine with a rise in GLP-1 [24]. These animal studies suggest a dual SGLT1/SGLT2 inhibitor such as sotagliflozin may provide even more powerful reductions in glucose, weight, and blood pressure in patients with type 2 diabetes.

Studies in humans have also demonstrated promising results with the dual SGLT1/SGLT2 inhibitor. In a recent Phase III trial, 299 patients with uncontrolled T2DM on metformin monotherapy were randomized to sotagliflozin or placebo in a 12-week dose-ranging study [25]. The patients given sotagliflozin (400 mg) saw a decrease in HbA1c, with −0.92 %, compared with −0.09 with placebo from a baseline of 8.1 % and 7.9 %, respectively. Additionally, significant reductions in body weight (−1.85 kg) and blood pressure (−5.7 mmHg) were demonstrated [26].

A small study of 12 healthy patients also investigated the effect of sotagliflozin on GLP-1 levels. In this study, subjects were treated with sotagliflozin at a dose of 400 mg daily at different meal times, leading to significant elevations in levels of GLP-1 and PYY [27]. Given the elevations in GLP-1, a subsequent study tested the synergistic effect of sotagliflozin in combination with sitagliptin, a dipeptidyl peptidase-4 (DPP-4) inhibitor [27]. In this study, 18 patients with type 2 diabetes were treated with sotagliflozin alone, sitagliptin alone, or the combination of sotagliflozin and sitagliptin. Compared to the sotagliflozin monotherapy arm, combination therapy demonstrated a statistically significant synergy in GLP-1 elevation [28]. In another study, patients with T1DM ($n = 33$) were randomized to sotagliflozin versus placebo, in addition to insulin, for a period of 29 days. In patients, given sotagliflozin, there was a significant reduction in basal insulin dose and HbA1c when compared to placebo [25].

In order to investigate the effects of sotagliflozin in patients with renal impairment, 31 patients with T2DM and an eGFR of 15–59 mL/min/1.73 m^2 were randomly assigned to sotagliflozin or placebo [29]. There was a significant reduction in postprandial glucose on day 7 in the sotagliflozin group compared to the placebo group. Of those patients with a GFR < 45 mL/min/1.73 m^2, the magnitude of the effect on postprandial glucose was maintained. There was also a significant reduction in systolic blood pressure in the treatment group compared to placebo after 7 days [29]. These studies show promising results of a new agent to use in the management of patients with diabetes.

6.5 U-300 Insulin Glargine

A recent addition to insulin treatment options for patients with diabetes mellitus is U-300 (300 units/mL) insulin glargine. This insulin formulation is three times more concentrated than the U-100 glargine, allowing for higher doses of insulin to be administered in a smaller volume. Pharmacokinetic studies have demonstrated a longer duration of action and more consistent profile with U-300 glargine compared to U-100 glargine [30]. The Phase III EDITION 4 trial studied 549 patients with T1DM randomly assigned to treatment with U-300 glargine versus U-100 glargine [31]. The patients in this trial had an average duration of diabetes of 21 years. The two treatment groups had a similar decrease in HbA1c at 6 months, and there were similar rates of hypoglycemia and adverse events. While this latest insulin formulation is an important new addition to the available selection of therapies used to treat diabetes mellitus, the use of U-300 glargine in patients with DKD has not yet been studied. Thus, frequent glucose monitoring and dose adjustment may be necessary for patients with renal impairment.

6.6 Delayed-Release Metformin

Metformin is one of the most studied drugs for the treatment of T2DM. However, its use is limited in patients with CKD with eGFR >40 mL/min/1.73 m^2 [32]. Recently, delayed-release metformin (Met DR), a new formulation that is primarily effective in the gut, has been developed and may be safe for use in patients with eGFR <40 mL/min/1.73 m^2. Met DR has a targeted delivery to the ileum, resulting to a lower plasma level of metformin for a given reduction in glucose [33]. A pilot crossover study randomized patients with normal levels of kidney function and CKD Stages 2–4 with type 2 diabetes to extended-release metformin (Met XR), Met DR, or placebo. Subjects treated with Met DR had lower levels of plasma metformin concentrations than patients given similar doses of Met XR [34]. Plasma lactate was not increased in any group. Further studies are currently underway to validate these findings and broaden the use of this drug in patients with renal impairment.

References

1. Kalaitzidis R, Bakris GL. Optimizing blood pressure and reducing proteinuria. In: Daugirdas J, editor. Handbook of chronic kidney disease management. Philadelphia: Lippincott Williams & Wilkins; 2011. p. 224–39.
2. Study of diabetic nephropathy with atrasentan (SONAR). https://clinicaltrials.gov/ct2/show/NCT01858532. Accessed 10 Mar 2016.
3. Evaluation of the effects of canagliflozin on renal and cardiovascular outcomes in participants with diabetic nephropathy (CREDENCE). https://clinicaltrials.gov/ct2/show/NCT02065791. Accessed 10 Mar 2016.
4. Efficacy and safety of finerenone in subjects with type 2 diabetes mellitus and diabetic kidney disease (FIDELIO-DKD). https://clinicaltrials.gov/ct2/show/NCT02540993. Accessed 10 Mar 2016
5. Scheen AJ. Pharmacokinetics, pharmacodynamics and clinical use of SGLT2 inhibitors in patients with type 2 diabetes mellitus and chronic kidney disease. Clin Pharmacokinet. 2015;54: 691–708.
6. Scheen AJ. Pharmacodynamics, efficacy and safety of sodium-glucose co-transporter type 2 (SGLT2) inhibitors for the treatment of type 2 diabetes mellitus. Drugs. 2015;75:33–59.
7. Polidori D, Sha S, Mudaliar S, Ciaraldi TP, Ghosh A, Vaccaro N, et al. Canagliflozin lowers postprandial glucose and insulin by delaying intestinal glucose absorption in addition to increasing urinary glucose excretion: results of a randomized, placebo-controlled study. Diabetes Care. 2013;36:2154–61.
8. Yamout H, Perkovic V, Davies M, Woo V, de Zeeuw D, Mayer C, et al. Efficacy and safety of canagliflozin in patients with type 2 diabetes and stage 3 nephropathy. Am J Nephrol. 2014;40:64–74.
9. Ojima A, Matsui T, Nishino Y, Nakamura N, Yamagishi S. Empagliflozin, an inhibitor of sodium-glucose cotransporter 2 exerts anti-Inflammatory and antifibrotic effects on experimental diabetic nephropathy partly by suppressing AGEs-receptor axis. Horm Metab Res. 2015;47:686–92.

10. Jerums G, Premaratne E, Panagiotopoulos S, MacIsaac RJ. The clinical significance of hyperfiltration in diabetes. Diabetologia. 2010;53:2093–104.

11. Cherney DZ, Perkins BA, Soleymanlou N, Maione M, Lai V, Lee A, et al. Renal hemodynamic effect of sodium-glucose cotransporter 2 inhibition in patients with type 1 diabetes mellitus. Circulation. 2014;129:587–97.

12. Ortola FV, Ballermann BJ, Anderson S, Mendez RE, Brenner BM. Elevated plasma atrial natriuretic peptide levels in diabetic rats. Potential mediator of hyperfiltration. J Clin Invest. 1987;80:670–4.

13. Thomson SC, Rieg T, Miracle C, Mansoury H, Whaley J, Vallon V, et al. Acute and chronic effects of SGLT2 blockade on glomerular and tubular function in the early diabetic rat. Am J Physiol Integr Comp Physiol. 2012;302:R75–83.

14. Oliva RV, Bakris GL. Blood pressure effects of sodium-glucose co-transport 2 (SGLT2) inhibitors. J Am Soc Hypertension. 2014;8:330–9.

15. Baker WL, Smyth LR, Riche DM, Bourret EM, Chamberlin KW, White WB. Effects of sodium-glucose co-transporter 2 inhibitors on blood pressure: a systematic review and meta-analysis. J Am Soc Hypertension. 2014;8:262–75. e9.

16. Malatiali S, Francis I, Barac-Nieto M. Phlorizin prevents glomerular hyperfiltration but not hypertrophy in diabetic rats. Exp Diabetes Res. 2008;2008:305403.

17. Peters AL, Buschur EO, Buse JB, Cohan P, Diner JC, Hirsch IB. Euglycemic diabetic ketoacidosis: a potential complication of treatment with sodium-glucose cotransporter 2 inhibition. Diabetes Care. 2015;38:1687–93.

18. Kohan DE, Pritchett Y, Molitch M, Wen S, Garimella T, Audhya P, et al. Addition of atrasentan to renin-angiotensin system blockade reduces albuminuria in diabetic nephropathy. J Am Soc Nephrol. 2011;22:763–72.

19. de Zeeuw D, Coll B, Andress D, Brennan JJ, Tang H, Houser M. The endothelin antagonist atrasentan lowers residual albuminuria in patients with type 2 diabetic nephropathy. J Am Soc Nephrol. 2014;25:1083–93.

20. Pyridorin in diabetic nephropathy (PIONEER). https://clinical-trials.gov/ct2/show/NCT02156843. Accessed 10 Mar 2016.

21. Efficacy and safety of finerenone in subjects with type 2 diabetes mellitus and the clinical diagnosis of diabetic kidney disease (FIGARO-DKD). https://clinicaltrials.gov/ct2/show/NCT02545049. Accessed 10 Mar 2016.

22. Wright EM, Loo DD, Hirayama BA. Biology of human sodium glucose transporters. Physiol Rev. 2011;91:733–94.
23. Powell DR, DaCosta CM, Gay J, Ding ZM, Smith M, Greer J, et al. Improved glycemic control in mice lacking Sglt1 and Sglt2. Am J Physiol Endocrinol Metab. 2013;304:E117–30.
24. Powell DR, Smith M, Greer J, Harris A, Zhao S, DaCosta C, et al. LX4211 increases serum glucagon-like peptide 1 and peptide YY levels by reducing sodium/glucose cotransporter 1 (SGLT1)-mediated absorption of intestinal glucose. J Phamacol Exp Ther. 2013;345:250–9.
25. Sands AT, Zambrowicz BP, Rosenstock J, Lapuerta P, Bode BW, Garg SK, et al. Sotagliflozin, a dual SGLT1 and SGLT2 inhibitor, as adjunct therapy to insulin in type 1 diabetes. Diabetes Care. 2015;38:1181–8.
26. Rosenstock J, Cefalu WT, Lapuerta P, Zambrowicz B, Ogbaa I, Banks P, et al. Greater dose-ranging effects on A1C levels than on glucosuria with LX4211, a dual inhibitor of SGLT1 and SGLT2, in patients with type 2 diabetes and metformin monotherapy. Diabetes Care. 2015;28:431–8.
27. Zambrowicz B, Ogbaa I, Frazier K, Banks P, Turnage A, Freiman J, et al. Effects of LX4211, a dual sodium-dependent glucose cotransporters 1 and 2 inhibitor, on postprandial glucose, insulin, glucagon-like peptide 1, and peptide tyrosine tyrosine in a dose-timing study in healthy subjects. Clin Ther. 2013;35:1162–73.e8.
28. Zambrowicz B, Ding ZM, Ogbaa I, Frazier K, Banks P, Turnage A, et al. Effects of LX4211, a dual SGLT1/SGLT2 inhibitor, plus sitagliptin on postprandial active GLP-1 and glycemic control in type 2 diabetes. Clin Ther. 2013;35:273–85.e7.
29. Zambrowicz B, Lapuerta P, Strumph P, Banks P, Wilson A, Ogbaa I, et al. LX4211 therapy reduces postprandial glucose levels in patients with type 2 diabetes mellitus and renal impairment despite low urinary glucose excretion. Clin Ther. 2015;37:71–82.e12.
30. Becker RH, Dahmen R, Bergmann K, Lehmann A, Jax T, Heise T. New insulin glargine 300 Units.mL-1 provides a more even activity profile and prolonged glycemic control at steady state compared with insulin glargine 100 Units.mL-1. Diabetes Care. 2015;38:637–43.
31. Home PD, Bergenstal RM, Bolli GB, Ziemen M, Rojeski M, Espinasse M, et al. New insulin glargine 300 Units/mL versus glargine 100 Units/mL in people with type 1 diabetes: a randomized, Phase 3a, open-label clinical trial (EDITION 4). Diabetes Care. 2015;38:2217–25.

32. Bailey CJ, Turner RC. Metformin. N Engl J Med. 1996;334:574–9.
33. Buse JB, DeFronzo RA, Rosenstock J, Kim T, Burns C, Skare S, et al. The primary glucose-lowering effect of metformin resides in the gut, not the circulation: results from short-term pharmaco-kinetic and 12-week dose-ranging studies. Diabetes Care. 2016;39:198–205.
34. Bakris GL, Mudalier S, Kim T, Burns C, Skare S, Baron A, et al. Effects of new metformin formulation in Stage 3 and 4 CKD: a pilot study. Poster presented at Kidney Week 2014, American Society of Nephrology, Philadelphia. 11–16 Nov 2014.